BIOGENEALOGY
Decoding the
Psychic Roots
of Illness

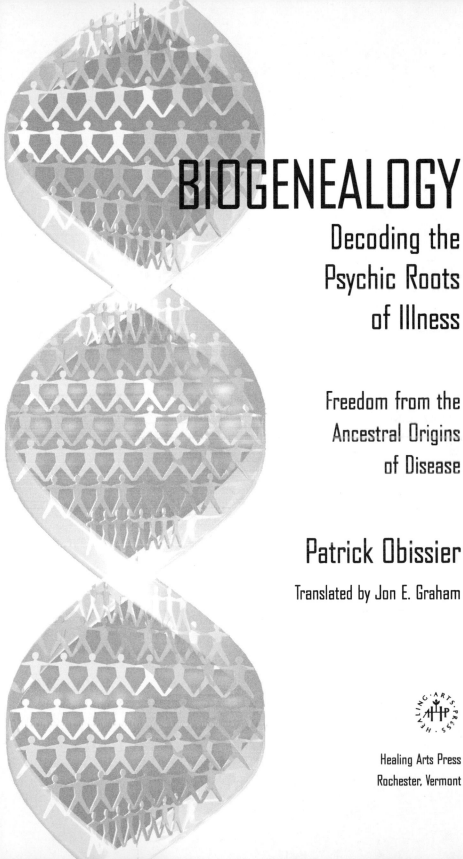

BIOGENEALOGY

Decoding the
Psychic Roots
of Illness

Freedom from the
Ancestral Origins
of Disease

Patrick Obissier

Translated by Jon E. Graham

Healing Arts Press
Rochester, Vermont

Healing Arts Press
One Park Street
Rochester, Vermont 05767
www.InnerTraditions.com

Healing Arts Press is a division of Inner Traditions International

Originally published in French under the title *Décodage biologique et destin familial* by Le Souffle d'Or, 05300 Barret-sur-Méouge, France
First U.S. edition published in 2006 by Healing Arts Press

Library of Congress Cataloguing-in-Publication Data
Obissier, Patrick.
 Biogenealogy : decoding the psychic roots of illness freedom from the ancestral origins of disease / by Patrick Obissier ; translated by Jon E. Graham.
    p. cm.
 Summary: "Reveals the psychic causes of illness and how to decode and resolve them"—Provided by publisher.
 Includes bibliographical references and index.
 ISBN 978-1-59477-089-0
 1. Medicine, Psychosomatic. 2. Medical genetics. 3. Genealogy—Psychological aspects. I. Title.
 RC49.O25 2006
 616.001'9--dc22

                                                          2005027847

Printed and bound in the United States at Lake Book Manufacturing, Inc.

10 9 8 7 6 5 4 3 2

Text design and layout by Priscilla Baker
This book was typeset in Sabon, with Bureau Agency and Agenda used as display typefaces

CONTENTS

FOREWORD

The book you are now holding, written by Patrick Obissier, is a book capable of talking to you about you. Without knowing you personally, it knows you! What kind of magic could be responsible for such a feat? The ideas put forth in this book work because they involve universal, transcultural principles that underlie every organized form of life.

From the information contained herein, you will be able to understand, integrate, and then put into use for yourself—as well as for others—the knowledge of how illness (infection, cancer) develops; how to prevent illness; and how to treat it. And you will come to understand how family memories play a significant role in the development of any and all illness. The views presented by the author are known by the umbrella term of *Biological Decoding*. Their articulation, supported with both theory and numerous case histories, extends from a global overview down to an examination of the smallest details. Nothing has been neglected.

To this complete work, which stands halfway between a clinical study and a personal journal, Patrick Obissier has brought both great power and a certain tenderness; he is both an artist and a scientist. As poet/therapist, he has opened the two "hemispheres" of thought so as to present his insights in a balanced way that takes the whole individual into account—both the thinking person and the intuitive, feeling person.

The power he brings to this exposition is that of the rebel confronted by the deeply entrenched views of a medical establishment slow to change its fundamental orientation. "It is not new remedies that people need, but gaining awareness of new aptitudes," he has said.

Patrick Obissier also possesses the sensitivity of the storyteller who has unearthed the appropriate metaphor, one that will allow readers, the patients, to evolve at their own pace on their own path of awareness. He observes, "In the cabins on stilts of our childhood, we seek for our past, greedy for the future." Patrick offers us the fruits of his personal encounters (with people such as Geerd Hamer, Marc Fréchet, Pierre Julien, and so forth). And he also offers us discoveries that have been ripened by reflection and his very active and joyful intuition.

These fruits, like the apricot tree of flaming hues at the beginning of the summer (a flavorful torch), are capable of feeding you, the reader, in a thousand-and-one ways. It is possible that, from these insights, a fruit will germinate inside you, just as it germinated within me, and then become a handsome, generous tree, replete with its offerings of good health.

I wish you happy reading and leave you in the good company of my old friend, Patrick—or rather, in *your own* company, of course! Because is it not your own unconscious triggers that you will be discovering here, recognizing and reappropriating them, to finally reconcile with the very thing—the sickness, the symptom, the disease, that particular facet of yourself—that is trying to tell you so many profound things *about* yourself?

But enough, not one more word from me! It is time to give the floor to Patrick.

CHRISTIAN FLÈCHE, AUTHOR OF

Mon corps pour me guérir, le décodage biologique des maladies
(MY BODY CAN HEAL ME: THE BIOLOGICAL DECODING OF ILLNESS)

Christian Flèche is a psychotherapist and a master neurolinguistic programmer, a practitioner of metaphor and symbolic modelling, and a highly regarded instructor of biological decoding. He also uses Eriksonian hypnosis, psychogenealogy, and memorized biological cycles in his work. Ever since the success of his books *Mon corps pour me guérir, le décodage biologique des maladies* [My Body Can Heal Me: The Biological Decoding of Illness] and *Le Roy se Crée* [The King Creates Himself], his workshops and seminars have drawn thousands of fans and influenced many therapists all over France.

PREFACE

*What great empire the mind has over the body,
and how often illnesses proceed from it. My cus-
tom is to race to heal the minds before I start on
the bodies.*

CLITANDRE, ACT III, SCENE 6, MOLIÈRE,
L'Amour médecin (LOVE IS THE BEST DOCTOR)

The Purpose of This Book

My intention with this book is to lead readers to adopt a tranquil
view of illness and destiny. I would be satisfied if they comprehend
that the way they look at these phenomena plays a large role in
determining whether they find themselves on the road to health
or the road to illness. But I am not seeking to inspire people to cul-
tivate positive thoughts that have no foundation—far from it.
This is not at all a new "Coué Method;"* quite the contrary.

Illness comes about, in part, due to a profound lack of awareness about the root cause of illness. Moving into the biological

---

*The Coué Method is the psychological practice of autosuggestion, named
after French psychologist Émile Coué (1857–1926), who pioneered it.

reality of the illness allows healing to occur by making it possible to see each symptom for what it truly is through an examination of that symptom's *meaning*.

Only through a full understanding of an illness and its symptoms is the road to recovery illuminated.

I offer many thanks to the pioneers Christian Flèche, Gérard Athias, and Marc Fréchet for their teachings, which were and still are sources of joy to me. Without what they taught me, I would not have been able to attain the insights necessary to write this book. Thanks also to these pioneers whose discoveries have enriched my life and work: Regis Duteil, Alexandro Jodorowski, Arthur Janov, Claude Sabbah, Françoise Dolto-Tolitch, Frederick Leboyer, Geerd Hamer, Georges V., Konrad Lorenz, Louis Angelloz, Liliane and Yves O., Milton Erickson, Olivier Soulier, Robert G., Pierre Julien, Josiane C., and all the rest. Particular thanks to Pierre Julien for his wisdom and friendship. Thanks also to everyone who read this book in its first drafts (M.J.C., C.S., J.C., and L.O.) and gave me their encouragement.

Thanks, finally, to all those who trusted me with their personal stories.

Warning: The contents of this book may conflict with your beliefs. They might also, by inspiring understanding and realization, prompt healing and other reparative effects. But the individual seeking a cure by means of biological decoding should be aware that not all illnesses have been decoded yet. More importantly, finding the causal feeling is one thing, resolving it is something else again.

INTRODUCTION

An Almost Perfect World:
To Dare Praise Illness and Destiny

Many will find it inconceivable that praise be given to illness and destiny. How is it possible to glorify unpleasant illnesses that cause suffering and handicap those whom they afflict? Why glorify a destiny that pulls an individual down a road far removed from the road he or she would rather take? Something can be praised only when its usefulness has been demonstrated.

It is the usefulness of illness and destiny that form one of the main themes of this book.

It has been with great difficulty, over what has been a period of more than ten years, that I have come up with a description of what illness actually is. In our culture, sickness is perceived as the result of an organic aberration, an inexplicable deviation from the norm, and thus something that has no value. Atheists cite the very existence of disease as proof positive that God does not exist. Furthermore, not only does humankind have scant appreciation for illness, we detest it.

I once felt this way, too.

During the past century, chemists, doctors, and biologists were all given the charge of waging war against illness in all its various manifestations. During this same time, seers, historians, astrologers, futurologists, and magicians of all sorts assumed the authority to speak about the meaning of destiny.

During a century of awe at the new possibilities made available by technology, researchers—in an essentially "masculine" way, spurred on by the necessity of coming up with quick and tangible solutions—gave little thought to the mental and emotional parts of the human equation, as if everything a living being believed, felt, or sensed was negligible and belonged to another, more "feminine" realm. However, in truth, it is the case that the two halves of an individual—the feminine and the masculine—are united in a journey toward the future, at every instant of life.

Doctors and most people today still consider cancer the plague of plagues, an insane and anarchistic process, whose origin is of diverse cause and remains a mystery. A paranoid atmosphere of defiance *against* one's own cells (*against* cancer, indeed, against *all* illness) thus prevails in the human psyche.

But everyone hungers for other, better answers. Twenty-odd years ago researchers in France and Germany, starving for the truth, had the audacity to look at illness from another perspective: by seeking the trigger mechanisms of illness in the almost immaterial sphere of "memories," or memorized information. What they discovered, and the cures that were prompted by their discoveries, could revolutionize the therapeutic arts and transform the world of medicine.

Between the discovery of germs by Louis Pasteur in the first half of the nineteenth century and the decade of the 1980s, nothing of overwhelming significance occurred in the field of medicine. Because germs were regarded as the culprits in *all* disease, the field of investigation into the genesis of illness was circumscribed. Relying on the scientific research they hope will invent magic weapons against illness, the "Pasteurized" researchers (those whose curiosity is limited by the conviction that the microbe is Public Enemy Number One) have ceased asking themselves, "What purpose is illness trying to serve?"

If illness were truly useless, it would not exist, for one of life's most stringent laws is that anything that serves no purpose disappears. Illness is useful, not because it helps limit the size of the human population by causing the deaths of individuals, but because it involves something entirely different, something human beings have failed to perceive up until the present.

The relationship that humankind has maintained with illness over the last millennium appears to have been a rather poor one. This was foreseeable, as illness is a very archaic process, a process we look at and analyse with a "modern" brain that is naturally oriented toward tangibles as well as the future, a brain that is quite capable of blinding itself to the reality of the past. It is inevitable that this natural antagonism between the archaic and the modern would lead to conflict. Most of us are unaware that illness and the programming of our lives (our destinies) have a meaning, a significance, and a positive purpose for the survival of each of us and each of our family lineages.

Before revealing how illness is useful and why it is preferable to work with it rather than fight it, let me first explain why the premature death brought about by an illness should not be blamed on the illness, but rather on the patient's incomprehension of the *phenomenon of illness,* as well as the misunderstandings of those around the patient and the patient's caregivers. New remedies for illness are not what humans need. Rather, we need new habits, and we need to make those new habits a part of our consciousness. If human beings understand the phenomena and traumas that befall them, they have taken the first step on the road to recovery.

Humankind has constructed all sorts of hypotheses about illness. Illness has been thought to be the work of spirits that have taken possession of a sick person. Or, illness has been believed to be a kind of punishment (the smoker is punished with cancer or emphysema for having smoked) when a connection can be made between an illness and the events preceding it. In other eras, the culprits were identified as miasmas, then germs, and finally, the cellular environment of the body itself.

However, *naming* what causes an illness is not the same thing as discovering its *meaning,* its true meaning, which legitimatizes it biologically. Sickness has a meaning, and it is not demented; it exists because of and through the context that gave it birth and contains it. By acting on this context, illness can be made to disappear. As a result, there is no longer any need to *fight* illness. The ability of an illness to reverse itself and disappear altogether is innate, genetically programmed, and merely dependent on simple stimulation.

It has become obvious that:

- All illnesses have a distress as their starting point, which causes "biological conflict."
- All illnesses begin upon receiving an order from the brain.
- As genes contain imprinted memories of ancient adaptations to old conflicts, all illnesses are genetic and epigenetic.

The Search for the Cause

Each illness begins with a specific feeling.

Arlette was assaulted one day. She tried to resist but could not manage to fend off her assailant. She felt powerless, and this was a source of great stress for her. Thirty years later, her son Jean-Louis felt equally powerless at the hands of school bullies, and this emotional tension triggered hyperglycemia. Hyperglycemia, or high blood sugar, helps an individual resist, because sugar is the fuel of the muscles, and muscles, among other things, are used to resist, fight, and repel. Thus, in this case, hyperglycemia was clearly the perfect solution, contributed by an organ, to help the boy's body fight and resist.

We find it natural that we inherit some of our ancestors' morphological characteristics and character traits. We might, therefore, also find it natural that our ancestors would pass down memories of what they "felt." By inheriting our ancestors' "souvenirs" of extreme stress, we are prepared for the possibility that we might encounter the same sources of stress that they did.

If we are in a state of preparedness, we can potentially react quickly to an illness and survive. To survive, even if sick, is to win time to procreate or—through our work, presence, or knowledge— to provide more help to our clan. If illness did not exist, we would die from the first extreme stress we experienced.

Because our ancestors live within us, we can find the roots of our illnesses in our family history, in our family tree. Then it becomes apparent that it is no longer the ailing organ that requires treatment, but our life experience and that of our family tree. Treatment no longer involves *fighting* symptoms by all known aggressive means, but finding the purpose of the symptom (what emotional situation pertaining to the "sick" individual does the symptom reveal?) to achieve a successful resolution of the illness.

The Genesis of the Discoveries

One summer night in the early 1980s, a young man was sleeping in a boat. Some gunshots were fired, severely wounding him; these wounds were eventually responsible for his death. His father, a brilliant German doctor who worked for a hospital, was sorely affected by this tragic event; several months later, he realized he was developing cancer.

The doctor was Dr. Ryke Geerd Hamer, formerly associated with the University of Munich and the University of Tübingen in

Germany. Following the death of his son, Dr. Hamer's wife died prematurely as a result of her grief over the loss of their child. Dr. Hamer, sensing that there must be some connection between his son's death, his wife's death, and his own cancer, was able to use his position as a doctor, researcher, and head internist of an oncology clinic to study his assumptions. He soon realized that a physical event can cause a shock manifested by a visible physical transformation in the structure of the brain that, in turn, triggers the manifestation of an illness. He decided to seek verification of his insight by asking his patients if they too had experienced any traumatic episodes before their illnesses appeared. As it turned out, all his patients had experienced a deeply felt tragedy before the onset of their illness.

This observation, which was later supported by thousands of examples, led Dr. Hamer to establish the five biological laws: the law of "biological conflict," which he called the Bronze or Iron law (this is examined in the following paragraph); the law of the two phases of illness; a classification system of tumors; a classification system of germs; and a law of quintessence. From this, he wrote a reference work on the subject titled *Foundation for a New Medicine* (Fondements Pour une Médecine Nouvelle). Dr. Hamer's research was based on his work (and that of his fellow researchers) with more than 31,000 patients over twenty years. His discoveries have been essentially confirmed today. They are the starting point for researchers, doctors, and therapists who are constructing a new discipline through the refinement, verification, comparison, completion, and sometimes the rejection of Dr. Hamer's research.

In the 1980s, hospitals equipped themselves with a new radiological machine: the computed tomographic (CT) scanner. When Dr. Hamer began examining brain scans made with these machines, he quickly discovered that a localized change in the brain always accompanied an alteration in an organ, and that there was always an emotional conflict associated with the onset of the patient's illness. He was able to help a large number of patients after the proponents of conventional treatment had given up on them.

Claude S. in France confirmed and furthered Dr. Hamer's findings. Gérard A. gave them their transgenerational dimension, and Christian Flèche managed to successfully combine them with Eriksonian psychotherapy. Other researchers made equally important discoveries by fine-tuning new related therapeutic approaches and by providing a deeper understanding of this or that aspect of Dr. Hamer's fundamental discovery.

We all know that to remove a bramble bush from a garden, it is not enough to mow it down or cut it with pruning shears. Only by tearing it out by the roots can we be completely successful in removing the plant. Likewise, if we tire of the continual reappearance of an illness, we need to wipe out the memory that gives that illness a reason to exist. This requires that we labor in our *inner* fields.

Those who bustle about in the moment see themselves as independent individuals and often have little awareness of the role they play in their lineage, the world, and the cosmos—the larger body of which the individual is but a cell. The individual lives as a leaf, not as a tree. The individual observes the immediacy of what is manifested, deprived of any insight as to its cause, because he or she has forgotten or ignores the past, the life experience of those who passed down the flame of life. Thanks to the recent discovery of the functioning of illnesses and their role in survival, allegedly impossible cures can be achieved, and human society can take a great leap forward.

It also appears that not only our sicknesses, but our life paths, our choices, our professions, our associative actions, the sports we prefer, the places we choose to live, our good luck, our bad luck, our fortune, our happiness, and our misfortune are also the consequences of and logical responses to old problems that have remained in a holding pattern in our family trees. For that reason, the meaning of illness and the meaning of destiny are dealt with conjointly in the pages you are about to read.

This book proposes a new way to look at illness through an exploration of the radical but ultimately logical idea that illness is a physical response to a past emotional trauma. It then takes the discussion one step further by exploring the idea that the extant illness can be either a result of a person's own trauma, *or* of a trauma experienced by an ancestor and passed down in that family's genetic code or epigenetic organisation. This construct is called "Biological Decoding."

To evolve, individuals have the capability to use their problems or illnesses to trace their lives back to the lives of their ancestors, much as the adult salmon leaves the sea to swim back up a river to a specific point on the planet and revisit the place of its birth. This is because *where* a person was born has a particular meaning, as does where the person's parents were born. By rediscovering the ambience of their origins—the context, the color, the "smell" of their conception—individuals can finally discover what debts they owe, pay them off, and choose the path most optimal to meet their individual, specific needs.

I forewarn the reader that it would be against nature to manufacture and hold feelings of resentment against our ancestors, or conversely, feelings of personal guilt, because whatever has been programmed can be deprogrammed. Every generation did whatever it had to do and, while the individuals of a previous generation may *appear* to be the cause of our problems, they are never guilty. We are able, thanks to our growing awareness, to cherish and heal the wounds of our ancestors, *a posteriori*.

Our road is also their road.

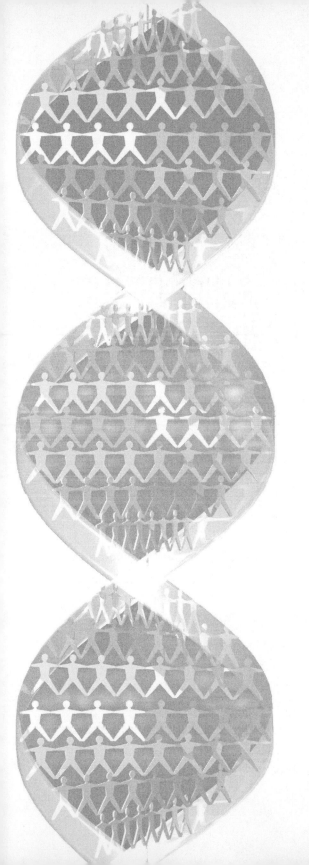

PART ONE
ILLNESS

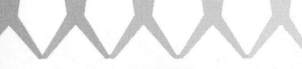

ONE

THE APPEARANCE OF THE ILLNESS PRINCIPLE

Genesis

There is a powerful force of attraction that combines scattered elements, such as the dust of shattered stars that was drawn together to form the earth. Might this force be what the ancients Greeks called Eros? Inside matter, whether it is in a gaseous, liquid, or solid state, molecules collide with each other at great speed, subject to forces of both disorganization and cohesion. Chemical reactions in the ocean produced the first "living molecules." Some of these living molecules began to synthesize chlorophyll and became blue algae; others did not and became various kinds of bacteria.

The combination of these bacteria and algae created thicker eukaryotic cells, which contained nodes capable of holding genes. After some of these primitive creatures lost the ability to practice photosynthesis, they were forced to feed on their birth mates and gradually evolved into animals. All these single-celled organisms possessed an almost eternal identity, because they divided into two identical clones, which would each then attain the volume of the original before again subdividing in two.

Sexualization, or When Adam Became Adam and Eve

Because these living creatures wandered about their oceanic environment, they encountered various hardships (extremes of cold and heat, falling meteors, pH changes, volcanic eruptions, the transition from a carbonic atmosphere to an oxygenated atmosphere, lightning strikes that carbonized and decomposed the elements in their environment, predation, and so forth), all of which could have engineered their disappearance. Thus, their survival depended on their ability to adapt rapidly.

These living creatures evolved thanks to brief and haphazard ciliary couplings (the foreshadowing of coitus) that allowed them to exchange pieces of chromosomes (bacterial coupling). Such chromosome pieces are like history books that are written as the creature experiences different ordeals and evolves in order to adapt to them.

But the evolution obtained by this means was far too slow. Once everything seemed firmly established, a new element entered the equation that prevented creatures from becoming imprisoned by habit, an element that forced them to move or change.

Nature perfects itself out of necessity, and sexualization was both a logical and a brilliant adaptive response. If two individuals are required to create a third, then the contributions made by each individual parent, in terms of information about its environment and experience, are doubled. The zones of skill (or adaptation abilities) possessed by each parent are acquired by the new creature.

One day (unless it was a night), Adam, a cell created by reproduction through schizogenesis, had one side (rib) that became receptive and female (this was Eve, the force that sets things in motion).

The two sides separated, the other side becoming an emitter and male. The biblical myth of Adam and Eve recounts the appearance of a male principle and a female principle from an androgynous Adam. Sexualization caused mankind to evolve quite rapidly.

Over the course of the history of living creatures, certain species have evolved and then regressed: asexual reproduction was followed by sexual reproduction before taking a step backward to asexual reproduction again. These alternations and variations were survival mechanisms. Some plant and animal species today possess both capabilities for reproduction, utilizing one over the other depending on variations in their environments (temperature, for example).

Certain living creatures can also alternate between being male and female. This is seen in the successive hermaphroditism of sponges, mollusks, fishes (such as the grouper), and amphibians. This observation allows us to grasp the ease with which creatures can evolve, regress, mutate, even merge with others that are dissimilar (chimerization, for example) to adapt to a problematic environment. It is important to this process that no scrap of knowledge ever be lost, and that any memory of form or function that proved useful at any particular time be retained. Therefore, all living creatures are equipped with data banks, chromosomes, and genes so that their descendants will be able to use an old recipe if circumstances call for it. Genes are the necessary records of the responses made by creatures to the problems they have experienced. They are testimonies to that experience.

And the Function Created the Organ

Just as atoms bond together to form molecules and remain bonded because this organization allows them to save energy, single-celled organisms combine to become stronger and larger. We all know how the whole is often more than the sum of its parts. The bonding association allows an economy of energy to be achieved. Multi-celled organisms form a cluster of agglutinated cells. Circuits are then constructed between the various cells of these clusters; these circuits are used by messenger molecules, ensuring communication between the different parts of the whole.

The universal law of economy again ensures the *specialization* of the cells inside the "multicellular individual." For instance, only *some* cells (those that will become testicles and ovaries, or pistils and anthers) are given the specific mission of dealing with repro-duction, just as in the hive only the queen bee has the right to lay eggs, while other bees take care of fulfilling the elementary needs of the community.

Another example: For a supply of food to be constant and less dependent on the moment, the physical organ of the liver was formed as an expanded part of the cell that formerly had performed the same function of metabolizing carbohydrates for absorption. The bladder likewise created itself to store urine, once there was no longer a need to constantly expel it. (Creatures needed to expel urine constantly for the purpose of marking territory, and as soon as this was no longer essential, the need to store urine replaced the old need of having to continuously expel it.)

Fins are specialized organs that developed to allow rapid move-ment. When marine creatures left the ocean for the land, fins became flatter and flatter through the evolution of fish to amphibians, then reptiles, rats, monkeys, and so forth, on up to modern humans.

Every new generation is slightly different from the preceding one. At the end of X numbers of generations, the liver is greater in size and consists of more cells, and the whole is equally larger. Over the course of evolution, these cells have evolved, through adapta-tion to their changing environment, in both the quality and quan-tity of their constituent tissues.

Tumors are a result of this phenomenon. We call them illnesses when they manifest in a way that is harmful to an individual, or to that individual's lineage over several generations. The universal law of economy also ensures that a cell that was reinforced during a specific period loses this reinforcement once it is no longer useful during another period. Bone lysis, atrophy, and ulcers have their origins in this strictly adaptive phenomenon.

An Adaptive Sympathicotony

The lifespan of multicelled organisms is greater than the lifespan of single-celled organisms because the cells that make up the multicelled organism renew themselves a certain number of times before that organism dies. The frequency with which problems can occur for multicelled organisms (the risk of death; being the victim of a predator) pushes these creatures to construct an adaptation system (faster than asexual reproduction) to permit the individual—and not merely its line—to increase its chances of survival.

These ultra-rapid adaptation systems are composed of an information storehouse and a triggering mechanism. All old experiences (remember, nothing that happened to our ancestors is ever forgotten), all the memories concerning the specific adaptation (ruse, combat, ancestral strategy, the maneuvering of a tissue, of an organ, of the body), are stored in the genes. The more recent experiences of the family line would be recorded epigenetically (thanks to the channels in the chromosomal regions, a sensible arrangement of the genes, the DNA molecules forming additional memories, and so forth)—in other words and for practical purposes, what we call cellular memory.

However, a triggering mechanism is required—in less time than it takes to say so—to search the genes for the old strategies and buried knowledge that will help the individual in the here and now. This triggering mechanism is known as the sympathetic nervous system, and it is part of the autonomic nervous system, which we will discuss shortly.

Sympathicotony, or the use of the sympathetic nervous system, gives an individual that is facing a threat to its existence a means of living longer. For example, in the event of a lack of air, a network of nerves and molecular secretions awakens the genes of the pulmonary alveoli. Their genetic expression changes; their cellular division is no longer checked, and will remain unchecked for as long as the problem exists. A tumor is thus a case of accelerated evolution. A tissue mutates in the space of several weeks, utilizing knowledge that its species has spent millions of years crafting through evolution.

Thanks to sympathicotony and the messenger molecules it sends to the hormones, neurotransmitters, and the immune system, the lifespan of complex creatures (that is, creatures consisting of several cells) is extended. So whereas sexual reproduction has already allowed a species to survive by incorporating a means to adapt more broadly and quickly to problems, the sympathicotonic portion of the autonomic system adds more resources that enable the individual's survival.

DNA is the elixir of long life.

From the Autonomic Brain to the Psychic Brain

Over the course of evolution, a command center was constructed to manage the different parts of the organism harmoniously for the individual's greater good. This command center is the automatic neurovegetative brain, or autonomic brain (automatic in that it acts independently of our conscious will). Every paleontological era has been characterized by new learning curves, an evolution of the relation between living matter and minerals. Each time, new layers of neurons are added and assigned to memory, the mind, and conscious thought. These new layers facilitate imagination, the construction of beliefs, and curiosity. The human brain gradually increased in volume around an emotional brain (known as the limbic brain), memorizing the incidents of excessive stress and constantly updating them.

The communication between different cerebral zones ensures that all thoughts, ideas, and words that are heard and all things that are seen can—depending on the intensity of emotion they inspire—act on all parts of the body by way of the neurovegetative brain.

Intense fear or other deeply experienced negative feelings create an emotional surge of stress that brings about a massive discharge of dynamizing catecholamines (adrenaline, noradrenaline, and so on). But these emotions and the surge they create could bring about *instant death* if no system existed to divert the stress caused by the shocks. The automatic neurovegetative or autonomic brain directs the energy toward a target that "sickens" in the tenth of a second that follows the initial shock, thus permitting the individual to stay alive. If the brain weighs around 1,300 grams and the body 55,000 grams, it would seem logical that the body would play a role in absorbing excessive stress. With the recent discovery of "minibrains" at the level of several organs, we could even say that these organs possess intelligence.

The Tennis Ball

Exert a horizontal pressure (F) on a body, for example, a tennis ball. What happens? The ball moves and does not undergo any deformation.

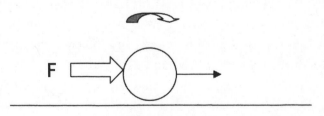

Figure 1.1

Now exert two identical degrees of pressure $(F + F_2)$ on opposite sides of this ball. The ball is unable to move, so the two pressures enter the ball, deforming it.

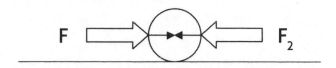

Figure 1.2

Similarly, with a living creature, when an individual finds no external liberating solution to the constraints it suffers, the result of the contrary pressures brings about an internal deformation, and the conflicting pressure is deposited within an organ. This organ does not react irrationally by doing just anything. It lends its aid to the body by intelligently modifying its own specific function (via an alteration of cellular renewal, mutation, atrophy, hypertrophy, hypo- or hypersecretion, and so on).

TWO

BIOLOGICAL CONFLICT IS THE CAUSE OF ALL ILLNESS

Emerging from barbarism is a slow process and as man is, geologically speaking, still very young, he has his whole future before him.

THEODORE MONOD,
Sortie de secours (EMERGENCY EXIT)

Every illness begins with a "cold phase," influenced by the sympathetic nervous system, and ends with a "hot phase." The cold phase is triggered when the individual experiences distress colored by a specific emotion. The lack of resolution for the problem creates and maintains a so-called "biological conflict." A compensatory chill will then establish itself. This moment is called a DHS.* In the cold phase, a so-called "cold" illness establishes itself in the

---

*DHS is an acronym for the Dirk Hamer Syndrome, named in honor of Dr. Ryke Geerd Hamer's son.

body. As this cold illness does not cause any pain, its presence may not be noticed (except in the case of motor or sensory paralysis, or a breakdown in secretion causing fainting or low blood sugar, and so forth). This cold phase often appears during a check-up, or a more targeted test (such as biochemical analyses or X-rays).

This cold illness (or cold necrotic phase of illness) enables the individual to avoid immediate death from an overdose of neurotransmitters or from a mishap that results from inattentiveness. An organ (and its cerebral extension) absorbs the greatest part of the stress so that the individual can survive.

The cold illness also gives the individual the assistance of a part of the body to confront a problem that the individual is incapable of resolving consciously. It is, therefore, a survival mechanism. (It is, of course, extremely difficult for the parents of handicapped children—those with muscular dystrophy, autism, Down syndrome, and so forth—to accept that their child's illness is a survival strategy, and I understand their objections. Some destinies are unfortunately quite tragic. The part of this book dedicated to destiny demonstrates how illnesses are archaic responses to problems experienced by our ancestors. I am convinced that our changing ideas about health will result in large reductions in the occurrence of these illnesses.)

▲

Given that the cold phase of an illness is precipitated by a stressful event that is experienced individually and felt painfully and deeply, the ensuing state of shock is a manifestation of what is called a "biological conflict." The word *biological* indicates that the individual's conflict is connected to vital needs: territory, safety, having enough to eat, being able to pay the bills, start a family, have friends and acquaintances, satisfy sexual impulses, and so forth. We are capable of creating biological conflicts for every cellular function in the body.

The incompatibility between a living organism and an external element (a toxin, fungus, poison gas, radioactivity, acid, or foreign body, for example) also constitutes a biological conflict. However, we do not manufacture an illness every time we feel stressed. It is necessary for a "seed of conflict" to have been sown at some point in the earlier part of the individual's life or that of the individual's ancestors. This is known as the "programming conflict."

The conflict that sets off the later illness is called the "trigger" and it is actually a resonance of the initial programming conflict.

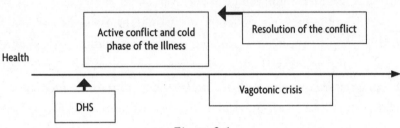

Figure 2.1

Here's an example of how this plays out: Anita lost her fiancé when she was twenty years and eight months of age. She went on to marry another individual and had a son with him named Aldo. When Aldo was ten years and four months old, Anita and her husband split up, and he was thereby separated from the girl next door, for whom he cared deeply. He experienced another separation from a girlfriend when he was twenty years and eight months (the same age his mother had been when she lost her fiancé). At this time, he began to experience short-term memory problems and to suffer from eczema.

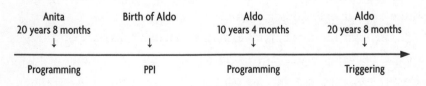

Figure 2.2

A small conflict generates a minor illness, a large conflict creates a major one. We are all equal to the extent that, if ten people share the same deep feeling, these ten people will suffer from the same illness. But we are not equal when it comes to *what* we feel deeply. Confronted by the same event, some of us create a biological conflict and some of us do not; some of us feel it in one way, and others experience very different feelings. It must also be noted that a small distress can arouse greater ones that are causally connected or linked by associations evoked by its information (like allergies). As an example, for a man: Learning the date of his retirement and the insufficiency of his pension can awaken conflicts of lack (how will I maintain my lifestyle and support my wife?). This kind of situation can affect the liver. A distress that is centered around feelings of devaluation (one is no longer capable of being the hunter who supplies food for the household), can result in decalcification. A scenario involving a loss of virility requiring some kind of booster can affect the prostate, a loss of direction can affect the surrenal glands, and lead to despair, and so forth.

A Very Useful Tool

As stated earlier, hospitals equipped themselves with a new radiological machine in the 1980s: the CT scanner. When Dr. Hamer examined thousands of scanner images, he discovered specific zones of the brain that were each in charge of an organ, or more precisely, a part of an organ composed of identical cells. The specific zones of the brain—the cerebral "command relays"—are located in the same place in every human brain.

Through his meticulous examination of thousands of X-ray images of the brains of those suffering from illness, and taking into account the marks, rings, and infinitesimal differences of contrast that had been thought to be meaningless up until that time, he realized that no illness occurred that was not accompanied by an earlier change in one of these brain relays.

When an organ is sick, it can be seen that a change had already occurred to its corresponding cerebral command relay; this change produces a specific X-ray image. It somewhat resembles what happens to an electrical coil when it experiences a power overload and loses its insulation, causing a short circuit. These altered relays were later labeled "Hamer's focal points" by doctors who went on to verify Hamer's initial findings.

Hamer gradually drew up a map of the brain that was based on scanner images of the brains of his patients and their case histories. As every organ has a specific function, the conflict that affects the organ has a relationship to this function. Hamer's cerebral cartography indicates the locations of the organ relays and the types of conflicts that affect them. It is now possible, with the aid of scanned images of a person's brain, to evaluate the person's psychic structure and conflicts. Furthermore, it is possible to get a very close idea of that individual's past, present, and sometimes future pathophysiological reality (and by the way, the locations of our cerebral relays are almost the same as those in the brains of our animal friends).

At this point, you should be starting to grasp how much less terrible illness is than we imagine it to be. The permanent correlation between the state of a relay and the state of the corresponding organ gives us a glimpse of a reassuring logic. Illness is no longer something that "just happens." Knowing that the body's organs and all illnesses are under the permanent control of various parts of the brain, we can begin to let go of the irrational fears that disease inspires in us.

The Transmutation

Given the intensity of a biological conflict, the relays affected by that type of conflict change, allowing an uncustomary electrical current to flow toward the organ they command, or, in any event, a current of a different intensity. The organ best suited to deal with a specific physical conflict changes its behavior in exact accordance with the emotional turmoil that the person is experiencing. (Person, from the word *Personare,* is from the Latin verb meaning to sound through, as in through a mask; or, in other words, something that resonates, that re-sounds throughout.)

Let's look at some specific examples of how organs are affected by biological conflicts. If *more* tissue or liquid secretion is required to resolve a conflict, the commanding organ creates more. A commanding organ, for example, may increase the power of the gonads to increase fertility, increase skin mass to provide more protection, or increase liver size to improve the body's ability to extract and stockpile, and so forth.

If *less* tissue is required to allow for the biological resolution of a conflict, the governing organ creates less. This can include less epithelium of the small curvature of the stomach when the individual feels separated from the desired fuel (love, strength, money, and/or other important things).

If the organ serves in a structural capacity or to facilitate movement (bone, muscle, tendons, and so on) it sheds mass when loss of prestige occurs, resulting in atrophy or decalcification. Osteoporosis, for example, is a condition that reduces the energy needed for the body to make bone.

If the organ is a container (a reservoir, a duct) of air, urine, blood, bile, and so on, the change could involve a reduction in the thickness of the container's wall to increase stockpiling or to facilitate the passage of these substances; the result would be micro-ulcerations (reduction in the thickness of a mucus membrane).

If it proves necessary to limit autonomy and movement because the person perceives them as a threat, the body's motor system may be affected by paralysis. On the other hand, if immobility or a restriction of the ability to make a gesture is the problem, the solution is an affliction such as tics, Parkinson's disease, or hyperkinesis, which will increase motor activity.

If the mind thinks it is necessary to reduce perception because the conflict has been triggered by what the person has perceived, the physical solution is a loss of vision or hearing. Conversely, if the conflict has been brought about by a lack of perception, the body's solution is to bring on hypersensitivity. At the time a DHS occurs, the illness is a survival strategy, but it is also a symbolic compensation.

The Role Played by the Kindness of the Breasts in Breast Cancer

At its onset, a biological conflict is a violent inner tension, a veritable internal hurricane. The absence of an external solution (recall the double pressures imposed on the tennis ball) creates the conflict and "internalizes" its solution.

Cancer of the mammary gland arises from a conflicted emotion connected to the idea of the "nest." One's nest is in danger. The nest is represented not only by the maternal woman, it is also the warmth and comfort of home, and the safety of the hearth, the spouse, the child, the child's friends, and/or the child's parents. A woman who, in the aftermath of a break-up or separation, is in despair about "making her nest" (no husband, no children) can manufacture a breast cancer if she has inherited this programming.

A woman experiencing a major problem inside her "nest"—for example, if her child, her husband, or another person, or even a cherished household pet, is threatened—views this problem from the perspective of a nursing mother. One of her breasts responds by creating an overactive mammary gland, a cancer, which is the body's solution to a problem she is consciously incapable of resolving. (The intracellular fluid of a breast adenoma is more nourishing than that produced by normal glands.) When a woman cannot find a satisfying solution to her conflict, one of her organs takes the initiative and creates the solution for her.

One hundred percent of the adenoid tumors in the gland of the left breast of a right-handed woman are due to these "nest-generated" conflicts. The event experienced and its emotional shocks (with their tones, undertones, and nuances) may vary slightly from woman to woman; they make up that individual's reality. A biological conflict, although it may be defined by carefully chosen words ("the nest," for instance), is generic, and it can contain almost as many subtle variations as there are people creating this type of cancer. There is an invariable structure, and then there is an "assembly" that is specific to each person.

The following poem offers an apt summation of the points we have been attempting to convey in this chapter:

The First Man on the Roped Party

Four mountain climbers
formed a tightly knit group.
They were taking for the first time
the southern façade of the mountain.
Halfway up their ascent
they were blocked by an unexpected difficulty.
Either they would have to attempt to scale an overhang
of crumbling rock, with the risk of the rope coming
*   undone*
and hurling them to their deaths
or they could retrace their steps.
Only an extremely narrow passage offered another
*   alternative.*
Immediately the thinnest of the four
threaded his way into the narrow chute,
and once he had made his way to the top of the
*   overhang*

attached a line to a piton
to enable the other three bigger members of the team
to rejoin him
on top of the overhang in complete safety.
Thanks to his devotion
he saved the roped team from certain death
and allowed it to reach the top.
It is the same for the body, too,
when it is faced by a specific problem
there is only one organ
that can provide a solution
for the body.

Small Causes, Big Results

The concept of a "problem" is naturally subjective. What poses a problem to one person does not necessarily pose a problem to another. Whether something is a problem depends on cultural and ancestral predisposition.

The active biological conflict that triggers an illness is not always obvious to the patient, because the conflict becomes eclipsed by the individual's attention and worries regarding the attendant physical illness. Often, the conflict is so pregnant and lasts so long that the individual gradually comes to identify with it unconsciously to such an extent that he or she can no longer distinguish it as separate.

For example, following the departure of her partner, Constance felt as if she did not have the energy to rebuild her life, to make a place for herself in a new setting. She was fearful of losing herself again. She created a Type 2 diabetes of steroidal origin. Constance had long had high blood sugar and, although she had eliminated much of the sugar from her diet, her blood sugar level remained high and even increased. (This sugar represents the energy and sweetness that was missing from her life.) Resistance had become such an ingrained habit for her (resistance to the idea of aging, to having to rent out half her house, to having to make do, to the bad omens foretold by the witch next door, and to the pleasure she derived from eating sugar, among other things) that she was no longer aware she was in a state of resistance. This phenomenon is psychologically known as "unconscious repression." Because one is enmeshed within a conflict, one can no longer see it, and one comes to believe that everyone feels the same thing.

The Nature of the Biological Conflict

If six different people *feel* the same thing when experiencing a shock, they will each manufacture the same illness. But one's ancestral history provides a prism that gives preference to some of the colors that pass through it. This is how the same event can be experienced in different ways by different people and thus produce different emotional reactions.

Each of us has inherited specific sensitivities from our ancestors. Furthermore, such sensitivities could be said to exist in harmony with the universe. (Every family has extra sensitivity to a certain health issue; there are eczema families, breast cancer families, rheumatism families, and so on.)

Given the fact that all family genetics and histories are different, when confronted with an identical event (for example, a wife surprises her husband in the shower with her best friend), the emotional reactions of ten different women would be quite different. To "amortize" the extreme distress, some woman in this situation might use the large curve of the stomach (this is an experience they cannot digest), others the bladder (the bladder is the organ which permits one to mark his or her territory), while others might use their colon (because they cannot forgive, and the woman involved was their best friend) to manufacture a polyp or a tumor. If their primary reaction is one of shock over the fact that they witnessed the betrayal in their own home, a woman might use her right breast (her first thought is of divorce, the end of the cozy nest), and others might use the retina (sight is the most valued sense, and what they saw horrified them), and on and on. But a woman who accepted this scene (perhaps she too had a lover and felt uneasy about concealing that fact) might not create a biological conflict.

Here's another example: A steady supply of food (from hunting, fishing, etc.) is just one component that makes up the stable environment of a group of people living in a balanced natural environment. But if, as a result of repeated assaults, the environment has become depleted, or if the people's needs (to wage war, support their sexual partners and children, buy cars, or build houses), outstrip the simple daily needs of their bodies, everything becomes more difficult, and nature and the ecosystems deteriorate.

When fishermen are faced with a smaller number of fish in their catch, they increase the size of their nets and the frequency with which they go to sea. When people are confronted by a persistent scarcity of food, and this scarcity becomes an obsession, they increase the size of their livers (the liver's nodules allow the extraction and stockpiling of more energy from food).

When Biological Conflict Becomes Commonplace

A traditional "cultural" behavior can both make the bed and facilitate the burial of a biological conflict. For example, in a family with a tendency toward self-depreciation, a biological conflict related to depreciation will be hidden (because self-depreciation is normal) to such an extent that the person in conflict is not even able to perceive it.

Women who were tomboys when they were young (either because their fathers wanted boys or because their mothers were humiliated by their husbands) have a tendency to manufacture breast or ovarian cancers more easily, and they have no hesitation about having the parts of the body that typically symbolize femininity surgically removed, in an attempt (unconscious, of course) to obtain the love of their parents and ancestors by becoming more "like boys."

A disagreeable emotional sensation can remain hidden quite easily when the event that inspired it has also prompted pleasant feelings. The person keeps the good impression in the awareness and conceals the bad one. For example, a girl who receives little in the way of tender, loving feelings from her parents might hide the despair and jealousy inspired by the birth of a little sister, who will steal her parents' attention, but who will also be a source of new joy to her. She will take care of her little sister and, years later, will not even be able to imagine that the arrival of her little sister also caused her pain.

Plants and animals also create biological conflicts, as we see in the following chapter. *But they do not aggravate their illnesses with fears and beliefs.* Humans, by moving further away from instinctive and primitive life, and by orchestrating and repressing things, have created additional opportunities for experiencing conflicts. Prohibitions, taboos, and beliefs constructed by the brain, as well as the fears generated by these beliefs, form a very fertile compost for illness.

Humans have set off to conquer the world with greed, the desire for power, the aptitude for murder, and belief systems (for example, that the white race is superior to indigenous races) that their enormous and still overly receptive brains have encouraged. Forgetting to live simply, in harmony with nature, they have sought to crush their fellow humans and, after cycles of repeated incidents, they have inherited destinies and illnesses without always inheriting the knowledge of how to manage their "wheel of life."

After three million years of existence, humankind has still not managed to emerge from its childhood, from its barbarous nature. Taming a brain that is rich with so many possibilities requires time,

29

countless turns of the merry-go-round around the sun, so that the causes of each element can finally be revealed and properly dealt with.

At the summit of the belief structure, the ideas one has about death may or may not give birth to biological conflicts. Words are the symbols for the things of this life, and those in positions of power learned very early how to use them to sculpt people's brains. With both the spoken and the written word, the powerful have created fears that allow them to control and subjugate. The idea of hell, a place of torment after death (which is based on no logical rationale), has enabled leaders to render their people docile. This belief feeds fear and allows imagination to prevail over reality, encouraging the appearance of biological conflicts. Another common fantasy or delusion gives individuals false assurance that they have some grip on the course of events and the lives of others.

Humanity's recent evolution has passed through several such episodes in relation to religion. The original messages of the Hebrew prophets were either "perverted" or poorly interpreted and their meaning diluted. The invention of original sin offered a contrasting model of godliness that had the effect of devaluing ordinary human life. Social hierarchies can be the source of the conflicts people create for themselves, as in the case of frustration, for example, when people compare themselves to others. However, the survival of the species requires order and organization, as order allows individual energy to be used economically so that the entire group benefits from it. Furthermore, hierarchies exist in the majority of all societies, whether they be plant, animal, or human.

THREE

UNDERSTANDING ILLNESS

If one believes that humans appeared fully formed on the earth (in accordance with the biblical myth) and not as a result of the slow process of evolution, it is much more difficult to understand the meaning of illness.

How are we to grasp the meaning of a kidney cancer (a carcinoma of the collecting channels) when we are ignorant of the fact that an ancestor of humans lived under water several million years ago? This ancestor was the fish, and from it we have inherited the ability to block fluid loss. When a fish finds itself stranded on a bank or a beach too far away to be pulled back into the water by a wave, its main interest is to prevent dehydration. In this case, the carcinoma prevents the loss of fluid.

Anyone experiencing a situation of being out of his or her element is like a "fish out of water"—in a hostile surrounding where they must adapt to a new environment over and over again. Kidney cancer may develop in those who had everything and then lost it, and are currently penniless and having to start anew.

How are we to realize the meaning of prostate cancer (*prostate* derives from a Greek word meaning "to protect from strangers") without understanding that the prostate appeared in the first mammals in conjunction with internal fertilization? With this type of fertilization, the spermatozoa must be protected during their journey inside the female's body to optimize the chance of an egg being fertilized. This is precisely why the prostate and the prostatic fluid evolved, to protect the spermatozoa during their migration to the fallopian tubes.

The biological conflict that involves the prostate is called a "semi-sexual abnormality." Connected to procreation, there may be an acidic relationship between a man and a woman; an uncommon sexuality; children who are not having grandchildren; or a problem associated with the traditional male role. The man who watches old age approaching with fear and wishes to show proof of his performance (he feels he needs to boost himself) in order to gurantee his male role, can, when triggered by an emotional shock, set off a prostate disease.

On the behavioral side, a man who has manufactured a hypertrophied prostate often demands to be a leader and wishes to have followers; this is the kind of person who has trouble getting his creativity to blossom. He would like to be considered a great sage and protector and to be recognized for what he knows.

The Four Families of Biological Conflicts

1. *Vital conflicts.* Vital conflicts concern the organs that take care of the individual's primary needs: oxygenation of the blood (fear of suffocation and fear of dying affect the pulmonary alveoli); basic fears with regard to not having enough of something (not enough to eat, not enough respect, not enough money, and so forth affect the hepatic cells), concerns regarding progeny (the loss of a child affects the gonads), concerns regarding

digestion (a tendency to brood affects the stomach), concerns regarding elimination (being incapable of forgetting a "sordid" experience or being unable to forgive affects the colon), and so forth.

2. *Protection conflicts.* When individuals have had their vital needs fulfilled and can "breathe easily," their thoughts next turn to ensuring their security. The conflict of the fear of being assaulted (which can concern the enveloping organs such as the pleura, the peritoneum, the meninges, the pericardium, the epidermis, and the dermis) can make an individual vulnerable to all sorts of arrows capable of wounding that person's integrity, such as an insult, an aggressive look, a disagreeable contact, an actual physical blow, contamination by a germ, or a sexual assault. Here we also find the conflict connected to raising children and taking care of those near and dear, which affects the glands of the breasts, an organ intended to benefit others.

3. *Conflicts of self-depreciation.* Once people's basic vital needs and needs for security have been met, their next requirement is the ability to explore; for this they need a structure, a skeleton, so they can move about. A person needs the support of a group to venture out alone (to hunt, for example) more freely. Here the individual exists in the context of others, and conflicts arise out of this. For instance, if an individual compares him- or herself to another, the individual may create a biological conflict of self-depreciation, which involves the structuring organs (certain parts of the bone, blood, tendons, muscles, and connective tissue), and this conflict provides a framework receptive to all the possible shades of self-depreciation (being dependent, being of little importance, or not knowing which direction to take). If self-depreciation occurs because the individual feels defenseless or unprotected, it is the lymphatic system that comes into play.

4. *Conflicts of relationship and territorial conflicts.* When the primary needs, the need for security, and the need to belong to a

clan and explore the surrounding world have been satisfied, the individual seeks to create a stable territory; inhabiting the same territory for a long time allows the individual to know it by heart and to obtain maximum benefit from it. To achieve a stable territory, it is necessary to be able to anticipate—to see and feel in advance. The individual now wishes to take pleasure from life and form relationships. In this case, the organs concerned are those that conduct information and blood, then certain parts of the digestive tubes, the bronchia, the larynx, the vessels, the channels, the nerves, the epidermis, the cervix, and so on.

A conflict accompanying this can be triggered by anything involved with what the individual considers to be his or her territory, which can be quite different from that of another individual's: a lion's hunting zone, a person's partner, the home, a parking space, land parcels intended for agriculture, the car, a cook's kitchen, a manufacturer's market share, a business person's clientele, a family factory, access to the sun for a plant, and so forth.

Different problems can arise involving these territorial conflicts: The individual may fear for his or her territory (there is danger in the air) or have a problem respecting territorial borders. The individual may feel resentment within, or be uncertain about, the boundaries of the territory. A person can also feel sexually frustrated, or experience the frustration of no longer having a territory. This is how our biological brains are structured.

Before the Chicken, There Was the Egg

A dramatic emotional sensation caused by an event is never the result of a rational and objective analysis of the situation; it is the resurgence of a very old conflict that emerges at that moment to live on the individual like a parasite. When a person reacts dispro-portionately to the importance of an event, clearly the emergence of an old history is involved. A piece of information is already inside and is resonating inside that person. Thus, an earlier suffering is expressed, one which the person is not aware of or has forgotten.

Later we see why the genealogical family tree carries, as if on a platter, a ready-to-think thought that is also a pre-packaged extreme stress ready to be bandaged. But what was there before the family tree? The ninety-one basic elements? God?

A Super Homeostasis

Inside every living creature, as within the universe itself, opposing forces seek to attain the balance necessary to enable life to exist. The force of the expanding universe is counterbalanced by the force of gravity. This is the yin and yang of Chinese philosophy. The phenomenon of life prefers neutrality and balance.

Also, and in the best interests of the individual, the part of the brain that governs neurovegetative or autonomic function receives hundred of pieces of information a second by way of the receptors that are located almost everywhere throughout the body. These receptors inform the brain of, among other things, internal and external body temperature; the internal hydric balance; the humid-ity of the air; light; and levels of blood sugar, proteins, salts, cho-lesterols, gas, and various hormones.

The brain then stimulates or slows down the activity of the organs and reduces or increases the size of the different sections and surfaces of the body, as well as their discharges and output. It is permanently adaptive, working on the inner spaces and push-ing the cells to exceed their functions as much as possible. This is what is known as *homeostasis*, the ability to restore or maintain a relatively constant internal environment in the face of the pressures from external variations.

But we have long overlooked the fact that what the individual *feels* is also taken into account by the part of the brain that governs autonomic function. The brain symbolically adapts one or more organs to these feelings. It is a kind of super-homeostasy! What the individual is feeling is given as much importance as changes in the environment or the status of the body's energy reserves.

The brain never gives useless or senseless orders: if the blood contains an abnormally high proportion of cholesterol, it is because this cholesterol will be useful somewhere; it is a response to either an old need or a present need. If the blood contains too many platelets, it is due to the brain's response to a need. When memory fails, it is in response to a need. When eyesight deteriorates, it is in response to a need. It is our task to identify this need and seek out its origin in either the present life of the individual or in the individual's family tree. If, because of an emotional shock, the need exceeds the normal capacities of an organ, the brain prompts these organs to change and adapt.

A need whose image is maintained in memory—an ancient feeling—is just as real to the brain as a need in the immediate present. An organ also takes action, especially if the *conscious* part of the individual is ignoring the problem, to deal with an old and hidden issue that remains unresolved. The road to health, as we shall see, necessarily passes through such a realization.

Once an illness's mystery has been dispelled, the illness ceases to frighten the individual. As an illness is actually the *solution* to a problem, it has a value. To get rid of the sickness, the problem that engendered it needs to be eliminated. Wouldn't the real symptom be the event that one is manufacturing anew out of bits and pieces of memory?

Why Wasn't This Discovered Earlier?

There are several reasons why it was not until the end of the second millennium that these biological laws were discovered (or rediscovered), and precise correlations between intense feelings, cerebral focal points, and illness were found.

The use of the CT scanner beginning in the 1980s made it possible to understand the process of illnesses. If the scanner did not exist, it would be difficult, if not impossible, to demonstrate the existence of the *cerebral* process of illness.

The rejection of promising hypotheses has been common practice in standard medicine. The World Health Organization has indicated that when the medical profession adheres to a particular doctrine, and a study comes along that contradicts the doctrine in question, that study will be ignored.

Hard core Cartesians attempting to create statistical correlations between experience and illness are in for a steep uphill climb, because the "event" that prompts the origin of a conflict may not even be real. It is possible for people to create biological conflicts out of virtual or imaginary tragic events, or out of symbols. Experiments with scanners have confirmed that *thinking* about an object brings about the same energy and blood flow to the brain as actually *seeing* that object. In other words, when it comes to cortical activity, enacting or imagining an action, *thinking* of a thing and actually *seeing* it, provoke the same response. (Imagine that you have just put some lemon juice on your tongue. Doesn't the thought provoke a reaction?) A woman who can't reach her son by phone after a factory has exploded in the neighborhood where he lives can make herself *believe* that her child is lying buried under mounds of debris; for as long as she doesn't know whether he is dead or alive, she can create a "nest conflict" that will trigger a breast cancer. Russian researchers have discovered that biological reactions can also be triggered in animals by saying out loud the name of a signal (but not actually producing the signal) to which these animals have been trained to respond. Further exploration of this observation could lead humanity far in discovering the origins of language.

On the other hand, when the biology does not work on someone in my immediate environment, it is then capable of acting on me. (For instance, with the intense thought/feeling "I can't let Mother see me," Mother will not have vision problems, but my descendants might.) We can also create conflicts by taking messages literally, or because the brain interprets something in spoken conversation differently than it was intended.

FOUR

THE SAME AUTONOMIC PROCESSES EXIST IN THE PLANT AND ANIMAL KINGDOMS

Because plants and animals are obviously part of the evolutionary continuum, they have adapted and continue to adapt to adversity with mechanisms identical to those of humans. The plant, animal, and human lines of our planet have all emerged from the same first living cells. They have undergone the same trials in the same environments and have adapted with solutions appropriate to their distinct natures (either with hemoglobin and iron, or with chlorophyll and magnesium).

The borders between the animal kingdom and the plant kingdom are more academic than real. There are astonishing species of carnivorous plants. There is also a rich array of sentient, motor, and sensory properties in plants living both in water and on land. Numerous species of plants have flowers that follow the sun's course through the sky. These plants close up at night, only to reopen in the morning; and after their stems have been flattened to the ground by rain, they will later stand erect again.

The Plant Lines

As with humans, plants must have all their biological needs satisfied. If not, one part of the plant steps in for the benefit of the entire plant. As the plant is anchored to Mother Earth, it is incapable of moving to a new location or having an external reaction, as an animal or human might. Therefore, its survival solution is essentially organic.

If a plant is not receiving enough light, the plant's "brain" triggers a survival plan involving a rapid lengthening of its stems, which climb upward in their search for light. This could be seen as hyperplastic, or reactive, growth. The stems carry fewer leaves (their primary purpose is climbing higher), their structure is richer in water, their wood is softer, and their conductive tissues let sap circulate more rapidly (as it is urgent for the plant to find light).

This tissue, which is different from customary tissue, is the equivalent of strongly invasive animal or human tissue, which can be described as tumorous or cancerous. The plant, having propelled its growth beyond what is blocking its light, finally finds the solar energy it is lacking. Thus it lives normally, thanks to the life-saving proliferations of its cells, which, in gardener-speak, are known as "suckers." After the crisis has passed, these stems slow their growth rate and return to a normal state (and their leaves start growing again).

Given that these atypical stems are greedy for energy, when they are too numerous, some of them may disappear. Fungi are invited to multiply to gradually eliminate the superfluous stems.

This sometimes takes place with the assistance of intermediary and complementary parasites (like the fumagin, a fungus that develops on olive trees due to the presence of cochineals).

The cells that isolate and protect the plant from outside aggressive influences (the equivalent of the derma, the pleura, or the peritoneum of the animal or the human) also step in if the plant has been bruised or assaulted. A plant whose branch that rubs against a wall or another plant when the wind blows cannot resolve this conflict by fleeing or taking aggressive action. Instead, the cells responsible for the plant's protection form a shield at the spots that are under attack. A layer of slightly different cells forms an isolated band that is thicker and harder than normal to increase the distance between its interior and the attacker (this is the same process that creates melanomas in humans). If the conflict is resolved or if the attacker disappears, these protective tissues become superfluous, and their regeneration comes to a halt. They remain in place and harden, or are eventually eliminated by bacteria.

Some plants can secrete toxic tannic substances for protection against predators. Just as the human being exposed to an uncustomary amount of sun begins to tan, one type of African tree protects itself from over-browsing by giraffes and other herbivores by making its leaves poisonous to these animals. Another kind of tree protects its fruits from the voraciousness of lazy apes by providing a home among its branches to ants that attack the apes by stinging them.

A solitary plant that cannot get itself fertilized creates the necessary conditions for a permanent regression that guarantees it a descendant, despite everything. This comes about through autofertilization (the equivalent of marriage between blood relatives), suckering (the plant's roots produce new, individual plants), or natural layering (branches and/or stems that curve down and re-establish contact with the ground or water, producing roots and a new individual).

A tree that has had a large portion of itself lopped off creates a conflict over the loss of its branches and of everything they potentially could have borne in the way of leaves and fruits. A hormonal sprouting provokes a large flowering (just like the woman who, during the conflict of the loss of a beloved individual, manufactures a cyst or an ovarian cancer that increases the estrogen rate to attract a male and ensure successful fertilization).

From generation to generation, plants acquire abilities they did not have previously (resistance to cold, to salt, to humidity, and so forth). This is known as acclimatization.

The Animal Lines

Animals, like humans, are mobile, and their problematic issues can be resolved in two ways: concretely, by outside reactions such as finding sustenance, a territory, or a partner; or by internal reactions such as the development of physical illnesses or behavioral disorders—madness, depression, or issues pertaining to sexual identity.

A separation conflict will provoke a dermatosis for a member of the horse family, the loss of feathers for a bird, microscopic ulcerations for an ape, and memory loss or cancer of the mammary channels for a lactating female dog whose puppies have been taken away.

Conflicts originating in the loss of progeny (for example, a litter of cats drowned by their owner because he or she doesn't wish to care for them) forces the ovaries of the mother cat to produce, as a survival mechanism, a super-ovary that increases the chances of successful fertilization to compensate for the loss and allow life to go on.

Among mole rats, the queen, when she feels the estrogen levels of her workers elevating, causes them to feel stress to inhibit their estrus. This clearly involves a behavioral solution that allows the dominant female, by maintaining the hyperspecialization of each member of her community (the queen breeds children while the other members gather food), to guarantee the survival of her tribe. Among humans, a woman who is dominated, rather than being a dominant member of her environment, does not have the right to have children; she may spend her time only with married men and accept the role of mistress.

Microbes can also adapt to problems. Those whose lives are at risk from exposure to intense heat manage to continue their line by encapsulating themselves (bacteria "in shells"). This protects them from the heat, and they go to sleep, waking up only when there has been a decrease in temperature. Like other animalcules, such as the miniature brine shrimp *(Artemia salina)* that live in saltwater lakes, they have found a means of putting themselves into suspended animation. The brine shrimp fall into a profound sleep when dehydrated and reawaken in the presence of water.

The white butterfly of Manchester changed its body color by becoming darker to protect itself from predators after the black soot of the coal industry there had covered its natural environment.

Animals displaying abnormal behaviors have, like · human beings, a constellation of conflicts. One conflict on the right cortex and a conflict on the left creates, depending on the nature of these conflicts, sorrow, depression, exuberance, sexual obsession, homosexual behavior, fear, aggressiveness, apathy, agitation, bulimia or anorexia, and so forth. With wild animals that live in a clan structure, some of these behavioral disorders have an eminently social role, in that they enable acceptance of the rules for life in a group or herd *without* creating illnesses. For instance, male wolves who are not the lead wolves become seconds or "lieutenants." Because they do not have the right to couple with the females, who are reserved for the strongest members of the pack, they become homosexual or attempt to have hasty couplings with the she-wolves of the pack when the opportunity presents itself.

The conflicts animals create reflect what distinguishes them as a species. For example, a sea turtle normally does not create a conflict based on a fear of water. On the other hand, a human or a bird is much more likely to manufacture a conflict regarding the fear of drowning, because their life environment is essentially that of the air. Exposing a hamster to smoke will not trigger lung cancer. But the brain of the domestic mouse (whose ancestors have experienced fires on farms) knows that smoke can mean death. If it is exposed to smoke, it triggers a cancer in the lungs that improves its ability to exchange gases.

Ill animals are protected from a certain number of complications that humans manufacture when they have equivalent illnesses. Ill animals do not have a wide variety of therapies from which to choose. If a spot on an animal's body is releasing pus or blood, the animal licks it or has it licked by a companion. It is as simple as that. The sick wild animal (and often the domestic animal, too) seeks solitude and hides away in a corner, rolling into a ball and patiently waiting for healing to take place. If the animal's energetic balance sheet (the relationship between its energy reserves and the cost of its repair) is in its favor, then the animal's infectious stage ends, and it experiences a return to normal health. Otherwise it dies.

Animals can resolve certain conflicts more easily than humans in the same situation. The laws of certain human clans are no longer biological laws but artificial ones arising from conceptions of society, gender, caste, church, or legislative assemblies. The conflict of loss (with ovarian cancer) that a vixen manufactures when she has lost her progeny rapidly resolves itself with the first ovulation that leads to her mating with a fox. However, a female human being who has lost her husband may not have the authority to begin a new amorous relationship. When sexual coupling is impossible for moral reasons or clan reasons, her conflict persists, and her ovarian cancer continues to grow.

"Domestic" Plants and Animals

Once plants and animals have attained a life of safety and security in a human's home, they start to free themselves and become partially emancipated from the rules of life governing the clan. But nature abhors a vacuum, so what has been discarded must be replaced. This social disintegration leads the plant or animal to merge with the unconscious mind of the human who is offering it this protection. As a result, there is identification, or mimicry.

Domestic animals such as dogs, cats, cows, horses, parakeets, ducks, mongooses, ferrets, geese, and so on, like the ornamental or potted plants that live inside the house, become a continuation of the brain of the master of the house, a supporting branch that makes it possible for the animal to reveal to humans what humans do not know about themselves. Our animals can take on our conflicts and create their corresponding illnesses. They sacrifice themselves for us and somatize themselves in our stead, in exchange for the food and shelter we provide them.

There is a new school of veterinary therapy emerging today that makes pet owners aware of their feelings and behavior. If, for instance, the owner of a horse is experiencing a hugely irritating relationship with an employee, one of his or her horses may suffer from a digestive disorder. This problem disappears once the owner, becoming aware of the aggravation of the relationship, lets go of it.

The sensitivity of plants and animals in this sympathetic capacity appears to be limitless. It has been observed that pets are capable of detecting their owner's pathological states (sensing a case of hypoglycemia, edema, or diabetes, for instance) that the owner is unaware of. Insect pests that swarm cultivated plants are actually helping the plants adapt to the physiochemical and energetic characteristics of the soil in a search for homeostasis and balance with the aboveground reality, which includes the conflicted state of the person cultivating these plants, with whom they are attuned. Insects, fungi, bacteria, viruses, and parasites can all be useful to the plant or animal continually attempting to reveal what humans cannot learn on their own. They are the zealous agents representing homeostasis and the ecological chain of life. While our legitimate and egocentric needs for an optimum harvest sometimes run the risk of remaining unsatisfied, they can offer opportunities to search within for answers that we were unaware we possessed.

FIVE

HALTING THE ILLNESS AND RETURNING TO HEALTH

For the ordinary person, the world is a battle-field; for the seeker it is a school; and for the awakened individual, it is a garden of play.

CHANDRA SWAMI,
QUOTED BY ERIC EDELMANN
IN *Jésus parlait araméen*
(JESUS SPOKE ARAMAIC)

What Becomes of the Cold Illness?

Most often, men, animals, and plants eventually resolve their biological conflicts. Small conflicts are often resolved rapidly, mere hours after their creation, because the situation evolved or the individual forgot them by passing on to other activities. Some examples would include conflicts of anxiety (one's child has not yet returned home); annoyance (one's boss is acting in an unpleasant manner); irritation (one's partner has allowed the dog to get up on the bed, one's husband is smoking a cigar), etc. In cases like these, the brain will trigger the reparative phase on the very same day or the next one. A person who has grasped that the cause of every symptom is a feeling and has a solid understanding of biological decoding can make a recently appeared symptom vanish almost immediately, once he or she has made the connection between this symptom and the feeling they had just experienced during whatever had recently occurred.

Major conflicts are often triggered by an extraordinary, unique, and limited event that cannot be practically resolved (what is done is done)." For example: "I felt powerless to save my dog from drowning." Or "I felt powerless to pull the driver out of that car before it burst into flames." Or "I can no longer walk with my colleague at work, with whom I worked with such ease, because he died." Although these conflicts are not capable of being resolved, they are automatically put into abeyance after a certain time, and a process of the automatic activation of the hot phase of reparation is set in motion, prompting great fatigue without warning and alarming symptoms. The person seeking to identify the event that caused it risks missing it entirely in these kinds of cases because the DHS and the emotional shock are from a much earlier period.

There are other major conflicts that are not easy to resolve: "My husband left me for someone else," or "My child has disappeared or died," or "I am ruined," or "I have three years to get myself turned around," or "I am nobody," or "I have been betrayed," or "I have only six months left to live," and so on. The cold phase of the illness will persist or intensify for these major conflicts that are often reactivated on a daily basis. A concrete resolution of the conflict is often not possible. Here a conflict can be resolved by going beyond it and by becoming aware of it with faith and fervor (I give up this unobtainable project, I understand that loving is not the same as owning another person, I accept what I have refused, I refuse what I have accepted, I forgive, I understand that I am not a victim but share responsibility, and so on).

How the "Hot Phase" Manifests on the Mental Level

Now that a solution has been reached, everything is subsiding. Whew!

How the "Hot Phase" Manifests on the Level of Neurovegetative Brain Function

The short-circuited brain relays begin repairing themselves with an edema that sometimes causes headaches. The sympathicotonia gives way to a pronounced healing. The vagus, endocrine, and immune systems, with all their transmitters, can be the intermediaries between the brain and the organs.

How the "Hot Phase" Manifests on the Level of the Organ

The cold illness disappears, either gradually or quite rapidly depending on the nature of the illness and the kind of resolution, thanks to the action of a hot illness. As in other areas of life, one illness drives out another. Quite often the cold illness has gone unnoticed, and the individual sees only the hot illness that caused its predecessor's disappearance.

The organ begins to repair itself so it can resume normal functioning. It then becomes the site of an edema as well, which may be hot and is often painful. What happens next can include the elimination of tumors by germs, encystment, calcification, or the reconstruction of damaged tissues by normal regeneration or with the help of a virus. When the cold illness has involved a breakdown of a function, or caused the function to be excessive, the resumption of normal functions takes place without the appearance of an actual hot illness.

When the repair of the organs is well advanced, an electrical discharge from the cerebral relay pressures the edema to expel its fluid. That this electrical discharge is part of a logical recovery system has also been overlooked until recently.

Healing takes place at the end of this reparative process. But quite often, a reactivation of the initial conflict while this phase is occurring makes the illness chronic. Healing can be prevented by medicine that methodically eliminates the exuberant reconstructions of the tissue. The brain, naturally programmed to engage in restoration during the hot phase, remounts an even stronger attempt to stimulate tissue activity to restore what the human hand has taken away.

Healing is a normal, natural phenomenon. The brain is waiting for information, good information, so that it can give the order to heal. This information confirms to the brain that the conflict has either been resolved or eclipsed.

Coincidences

We are rarely aware that the "hot disorders" (the anginas, pains, colds, infections, inflammations, illnesses ending in -*itis* such as cystitis and nephritis) have their onset on the heels of a feeling of mental soothing. The period of mental soothing is best described as the resolution or cessation of the initial emotional trauma (which caused the cold phase of the physical response in the first place). When we *do* happen to notice that we are experiencing this mental soothing, it is usually to draw the bitter and perhaps too hasty conclusion: "I always feel great right before I get sick!" ("Getting sick" in this case means coming down with the "hot," restorative phase of the illness.)

It is hard to accept the idea that a soothing process could be the cause of a hot illness or the hot phase of an illness, as it seems totally illogical. But this is, in fact, what is happening. The simple fact is that we are unaware that we had a discreet, hidden, cold illness to eliminate.

In this chapter we learn that illness is eliminated on orders from the brain, which indicates that the illness is no longer serving a useful purpose. It becomes apparent that illness is a reversible process, and those who understand how to trigger healing will no longer be perpetual victims but decisive, determined, proactive participants in their own recovery. When we can see and understand that microbial activity is a necessary and restorative process of the body, our ancient fears will vanish.

Illnesses are our "jokers" that allow us to carry on despite having gone astray and made mistakes. No one really has grounds for glorifying the proposition that he or she owes health and vitality to a quality diet, because, as we see in the following chapters, illnesses are programmed and can surge up without warning despite all the dietetic and hygienic precautions we might take.

Here is an example of the way a biological conflict can manifest as a particular illness: Robert fought in the Algerian War while his brother managed the family business, which, in fact, was something that Robert himself had always aspired to do. This caused Robert to feel resentment, and consequently his bile ducts became ulcerated. When Robert completed his military service he rejoined the family company, and his resentment vanished. He came down with hepatitis, which repaired his bile ducts. Today he is happy and healthy and enjoying a fruitful old age.

The Eclipsing of a Conflict

In Algiers, Fatima, raised in a modern milieu, married a young man who brought her to live with him, his parents, and his sisters on the fourth floor of an apartment building. For many months, Fatima tried to persuade her husband to rent an apartment somewhere else for just the two of them. Nothing doing. Seven months after a sharp quarrel about this, Fatima began feeling tingling in her legs; shortly thereafter she began finding it harder to walk. Two years later she consulted a neurologist, who diagnosed her with multiple sclerosis.

Fatima had created a conflict (iatrogenesis) around the idea of becoming paralyzed and, in the weeks following her diagnosis, she truly became paralyzed. One evening her home was invaded by terrorists, and this new conflict of fear suspended her former conflict (her inability to push her husband out of his nest). She was able to walk with difficulty until the terrorists left. This is the operative power of the psychological brain on bodily function. One conflict can truly eclipse another.

The Transition to Chronic

One conflict may include several aspects, several strong emotions, and when all these essential aspects have been dealt with, the cure is complete.

The chronic state of an illness is due to the fact that the patient is once again faced by its causal problem (its resolution was insufficient) or has generated new, small conflicts around the illness. The old culture of illness ensures that, when a crisis is upon us, we quickly lose patience and interpret the phenomenon negatively. We quickly come into conflict with our illness.

Emotional suffering is then added to physical pain. This is why, although this survival mechanism with its two-phase illness (hot and cold) is remarkably simple, humans can have great trouble getting better. Their fear of not getting healed actually helps prevent healing.

The Duration of the Hot Reparative Phase

There is a Latin saying, *Venit morbus eques, suevit arbire pedes,* that means, "Illness comes in on horseback and leaves on foot."

Edema, inflammation, fever, and infection arrive at a gallop once the conflict has been resolved, but they take much longer to leave. Repairing an organ and its cerebral relay takes time. The duration of the hot illness depends on the nature of the cold illness and its extent.

So it is necessary to wait. The duration of this phase also depends on the patient's resources (energy, understanding of what is happening, certainty of being cured, serenity surrounding the patient). For healing to occur, the reparative phase must run its full course to the very end, which is when scar formation occurs. But when the conflict is reactivated, new conflicts appear, or some antireparative treatments are used that balance out the symptom, and the illness becomes chronic.

In other cases cures are almost immediate.

But some basic questions stand out. What is a cure? The momentary disappearance of the symptom? Or the profound conversion of the individual that eliminates the sensitivity to the conflicts that once possessed him or her? Is a cure the disappearance of fear? What is the identifying sign of a person in good health? Is it an ability to be present in the here and now and fully tuned in to the world?

Examples of Reparative Phases

A sinus cold is the hot phase that reconstructs the nasal mucous membrane after the ulceration caused by the cold phase. Otitis removes a tumor from the middle ear. A pulmonary infection eliminates tumors from the pulmonary alveoli. Hepatitis rebuilds biliary ducts that have been ulcerated. Eczema is one phase in the process of restoring the epidermis. Tendonitis is a phase in the rebuilding of a tendon. Rheumatism is a phase in the repair of a bone or joint.

Epidemics

The memory of recent Western infectious epidemics such as cholera, tuberculosis, and Spanish influenza (at the end of World War I) has solidly anchored the idea that germs are responsible for death and misfortune. It is, however, always through an evident collective conflict or by a concealed collective emotion that the epidemic process begins. The more people are concerned with the same problems, the more the same emotional shock is shared. Conflicts are collective. Put yourself in the shoes of the quiet inhabitants of a village that has just been invaded by Vikings. What would the inhabitants be feeling? They would be terrified of dying.

Collective alarm is the origin of epidemics, colds, flu, and bronchitis, to cite only a few afflictions. At the end of the year, the days are quite short, and natural light (the symbol of the protective father) is at its minimum. At this time, people are uneasy and in conflict, without necessarily being aware of the source of their anxiety. With the lengthening of the days there is a progressive distancing from the sense of death's proximity, as all living creatures are nourished directly or indirectly by solar energy.

With the resolution of conflicts, once the danger has passed and people are feeling secure again, the natural alleviation of the conflict automatically triggers the transition of an illness from the cold phase to the hot phase. Other soothing factors, including sociological ones, can be decisive.

The worldwide epidemic of the Spanish flu (which was responsible for between ten and twenty-five million deaths) began in April 1918 and ended in 1919 concurrently with the calm that preceded the cessation of hostilities and followed the end of the war. More people died from the flu than on the battlefields, because the conflict that triggers flu is fear about one's territory and fear for one's reputation.

To cite another example: In the late 1960s in France, the Asiatic flu was responsible for 18,000 deaths, 80 percent of which occurred in persons older than sixty-five years. However, when the social upheavals of May 1968 began to be incorporated into the body politic, the populace could see that the basic structure of society would remain unchanged, and their established rights and expectations (retirement systems, among other things) were safe. At that point, the disease began to abate.

Because the tuberculosis epidemics of the fairly recent past have affected the members of many of our families, this disease deserves a brief examination. The microbe discovered by Koch was charged with being the sole cause of the disease, as the cold phase of this ailment was never detected. Only individuals creating a biological conflict out of the fear of death (their own death, that of their nearest and dearest, that of beloved ancestors), or from the fear of suffocation (of course they would have to be carriers of the Koch bacillus as well), would actually go on to develop a case of pulmonary tuberculosis. Someone who is a carrier of the Koch bacillus but is *not* manufacturing a conflict does not create this illness.

The process occurs as follows: The fear-of-death conflict triggers one or more tumors in the pulmonary alveoli (which often go unnoticed). The biological response consists of the creation of additional pulmonary alveoli, which improve oxygen absorption so that the individuals have more energy to use in the battle against the threat.

Then, when people have calmed down (because the danger no longer exists, the invader has left, the demobilization of the army has been decreed, and so on), and the feelings generated by the fear of death have subsided, the normal rate of air absorption by the lungs is sufficient. The exceptionally large alveoli now have to disappear (because they are energy hogs), and the Koch bacilli break down and sweep away the now-useless tissue—that of the tumor, and only of the tumor. This heralds the advent of the coughing, spitting, nocturnal sweating, and fatigue that accompany numerous repairs.

This hot phase is a delicate period, because the belief that the illness is fatal reactivates the fear-of-death conflict. The reactivation of the conflict brings a halt to the tubercular infection, which gives the sufferer the impression of a remission. However, in reality, a new tumor is being introduced, or the first one is being reactivated. When the halt of the infection is confirmed, the individual calms down again, thus resolving the conflict and starting up the infection (the hot phase) again.

This is how the vicious circle of a chronic disease is established. The exhaustion it causes can lead to an individual's death while the person is going through the reparative phase, especially if the loss of protein (caused by the constant need to expectorate that is one of the symptoms of this stage of the illness) is not replaced by a sufficiently rich diet.

This should make it clear how people can die as a result of ignorance when they are just a few steps short of being healed, just like a long-distance runner who collapses a hundred yards from the finish line.

Allergies: Defensive Combinations

At the time a dramatic event occurs, the brain records one or more bits of information about the setting of this drama (just as a navigator takes readings to calculate a position), so that a physical response can be fashioned instantly in the event that similar information is perceived in the future.

Any extreme stress experienced when, for example, "it is 4:00 A.M., it is night, it is raining, and the smell of wet lavender is in the air" produces the following equation: 4:00 A.M., rain, lavender = extreme stress. This ensures that the presence of any *one* of these elements would be capable of triggering excessive stress as an emotion.

Rupert Sheldrake explains that a rooster goes to the rescue of hens in response to their cries of distress, but does not move if it only *sees* them in distress through a soundproof window (*A New Science of Life,* Rochester, VT: Inner Traditions, 1994). So while we all have five senses at our disposal to give us information, each of us uses one of these senses (sight, hearing, touch, smell, and taste) in preference to the other four. In response to a stressful event (Father is leaving Mother), a child's brain memorizes something unique in conjunction with the stressful event: one child remembers the smell of coffee; another remembers the song that happened to be playing on the radio; a third recalls the pollen that was falling from the plane trees.

This is why an external trigger can produce an emotional reaction. The elements present when the emotion was initially felt become, for that person, meaningful stimuli.

And if later this same stimulus is present in the individual's environment, the cold illness corresponding to the conflictive emotion is triggered, followed by its hot reparative phase, in sometimes impressive fashion (hives, malaise, coma, asthma, edema, and so on). The intensity of the allergic crisis is naturally proportional to the significance of the programming conflict.

An allergy to parsley can have its origins in a genealogical memory of an attempted abortion (in the past, parsley was a key ingredient in inducing an abortion). An allergy to iodine might be due to the memory of fear caused by diving into the ocean. It is neither the parsley nor the iodine nor any other allergen that is the objective cause of the exaggerated reactions of the organs, but what the allergen signifies to the person involved, either out of his or her own personal life story or one from the family tree.

Every individual receives an "album of souvenirs" at conception in which are recorded the potential dangers that determine the person's tendency to feel one way as opposed to another. Some people are territorial and extrasensitive to their space, others are more sensitive to aggression, others to self-depreciation, and so

on. Therefore, the majority of "pathological" allergies to identified allergenic agents are due, to borrow Jung's formulation, to
synchronicities—in other words, to the conjunctions of events and
things that have no causal connections.

Some illnesses are triggered by spatial stimuli (elements from
the initial setting, such as a smell, the temperature, and so forth),
and others are triggered by temporal stimuli (individual and universal cycles, hours, seasons, the first week of every September,
an anniversary date). But time can specify space: a point in time
(between 8:00 and 9:00 A.M. every July 15, for example) is also
a point that can describe a position. Thus, stimuli can be either
spatial or temporal.

In fact, all illnesses function on the principle of allergies. They
are programmed by excessive stress and triggered later by spatiotemporal stimuli that bring these feelings of great stress "back to
mind."

On Miracles (from the Latin *Mirus,* "Amazing")

Now that we know a biological conflict is the footbridge between
sickness and health, and that it is theoretically possible to reverse
the process, we can understand what, historically, have been known
as "miracle cures." All the miracle cures recorded throughout history are more easily explained.

The most common miracles are, in fact, those involving "cure"
of the hot illnesses—that is to say, the illnesses that repair the body,
whose biological destiny is to disappear of their own accord. This
observation does not diminish the worth of healing protocols, without which ill people would remain stuck in an unstable balance
between the hot and cold phases, or in the middle of the reparative
phase, or during the scar-formation phase at the end of the illness.

The most extraordinary cures are of the cold diseases, which
arise following a realization that has been intentionally prompted

by the therapist. But each one of us, every time we resolve this or that conflict, triggers a biological reaction that might be amazing to an outside observer.

After surgical measures (useful or superfluous) have been taken, after medical treatments have been prescribed (essential, helpful, or useless), if the individual is healed, it is because the conflict was resolved beforehand and the roots of the illness were eradicated. The ability to heal is ever-present in the body, but it cannot reveal itself completely. Healing depends on the decisions the patient makes, the patient's wisdom and willingness to accept help, and the patient's ability to abandon the outdated beliefs of those around him or her and to live in the here and now.

WHY ILLNESS? WHY NOT ANGEL KISSES?

The need for a system that can provide ultrarapid assistance to the body when it is in difficulty has led to what we call illness. Without illnesses, which are the jokers in life's deck, our life expectancy might equal that of insects. We need protection, life preservers, and a balancing pole to reach the end of our journey. What could offer more security than to be the carrier of thousands of protection systems? To carry one's guardian angel within, rather than having a potential protector who might be far away when needed, is clearly proof of the great intelligence of life.

An illness is an organ that mutates; it performs differently than it did before, or differently from what it is supposed to do normally. The frog has turned into a bull. The bull has transformed into a frog. The organ that is the most logically capable of helping the body says to itself: "I will make more cells (a tumor)" or "I will get rid of cells and create an ulcer" or "I will accelerate or put the brake to this function" or "I will block or reduce the production of this secretion," and so on.

An organ that malfunctions or becomes diseased deals three trump cards to the body it inhabits:

1. The immediate discharge of the extreme stress on a receptive organ prevents the body from dying as a result of an overdose of stress hormones, vasoconstriction, or even the kind of extreme distraction that can cause an individual to ignore potentially fatal situations. An answer has been found, survival is possible, and hope is reborn.

2. The modification of an organ or function brings something to the person in conflict (sugar for fighting, water to avoid dehydration, more air, more X hormone, more Y hormone, for instance). This is the "biological meaning" of the illness.

3. The illness indicates the existence of a programming conflict located in the first part of an individual's life or in the lives of the individual's ancestors, and it offers the individual the chance to become aware of this hidden extreme stress. It offers an opportunity for the mindful individual to "cleanse" his or her childhood and to treat the wounds of the individual's family tree.

Let's look at some specific examples that show us how an illness can be an asset. Corinne was a thirty-three-year-old accountant. Her employer abruptly fired her, and she found herself without resources. She felt an urgent need to do something quickly about this troubling situation. Her thyroid gland "exceeded" its normal function by creating a nodule that would secrete an additional amount of thyroid hormone. The extra hormone transformed her into a dynamo, which enabled her to continue her hunt for a new job more efficiently. Her friends nicknamed her "Speedy." Her mother, too, had experienced times of urgent necessity during an earlier part of her life.

Annie was fifty years old, and quite maternal, just like her mother. She realized that her daughter, living on the other side of town, was in great danger from her abusive husband, but she did not know what she could do to help her. Because she was at a loss as to what steps to take, she experienced a biological conflict. This meant that one of her organs would have to supply an archaic answer.

The sole organ that is biologically intended to help someone other than its owner is the breast, which is designed to feed the child, the spouse, and even, in the case of Amazon women, little pigs. Annie's left breast created a more effective extra gland (it was no longer a question of feeding a baby) that we call cancer. This new tumorous gland is capable of providing a more nutritious kind of milk than a normal mammary gland. This was the solution that the organ came up with for an individual feeling an urgent need to help her child.

Of course, this is a very archaic kind of response, as the daughter obviously could not nurse at her mother's breast. But because one of Annie's body's organs was offering a solution, her mental stress could subside somewhat, and Annie could continue living under a stress load that was physically tolerable.

George was thirty-six. Laid off during a downsizing of personnel, he experienced an enormous sense of self-devaluation. Then his fiancée left him, intensifying his low self-esteem. In nature, the constant search for the most economical path ensures that everything that no longer serves a useful purpose disappears. A living organism cannot nourish an organ it feels to be superfluous.

The support organs (bones, muscles, tendons) are the fuses that blow when the individual feels ineffective or useless in this or that domain of life. The shoulder, for instance, is inevitably chosen by the body to deal with conflicts concerning taking action, working with the arms, and taking someone "under one's wing." When George was laid off and his fiancée left him, he felt that he was no longer of any value, because he believed that he could no longer shoulder a job or a relationship successfully. His body thus decided to save energy by ceasing to give the correct food to the ineffective and useless organs, which would be erased through decalcification. The energy and calcium thus saved would be spent on other organs. The cold phase of an illness involves the decalcification of an organ perceived as ineffective, permitting the body to survive throughout the duration of the conflict, until such time as the conflict is resolved.

Anne Marie was forty-seven. She worked hard every day to feed her family and had to deal with her eldest son, who was violent by nature and beat her daily. She was skeletally thin and exhausted, but she was also stoic and refused to denounce her son. One night when she was subjected to a particularly violent assault, she became paralyzed on one side, which affected her ability to talk. This would turn out to be her salvation. The living hell of her life that she was not able to escape otherwise was brought to an end, thanks to her paralysis.

She had made every effort to keep everything inside and not reveal to others what was happening, but, by becoming paralyzed, she forced those around her to act. Her son changed his ways, and one of Anne Marie's adult daughters brought Anne Marie to live with her, enabling her to begin a second life in which she was cherished and protected. The biological meaning of paralysis is to force the individual to put himself or herself "out of danger" when the biological conflict involves a dangerous move or a choice between love and duty that the individual finds it impossible to make.

Josephine was a fifty-two-year-old woman who was adopted at birth and given the name of her adoptive mother. She was then taken back by her birth mother, who, at that time, gave her the name of her grandfather. Her mother remained unmarried all her life, serving her father as a secretary and maid. Josephine never knew the identity of her father, still missed her adoptive mother, didn't know who she really was, and didn't know how to mark out her own territory. She felt like someone whose "rear end is hanging between two chairs."

During all those years marked by conflicted feelings, she had an ulcer on her lower rectum. This organ is the symbolic organ of identity and governs the fear of being abandoned and left like a broken-down car on the side of the road. When Josephine married, she became the owner of a beautiful house, and this resolved her identity conflict ("I am not like the others"). Subsequently her rectum healed, with hemorrhoidal bleeding symbolic of the way she was marking off her territory, based on her great need to establish her identity. She had to resort to an operation to help finish this reparative phase because the extensive nature of the required repair was alarming.

Life demands a solution to every problem. When the individual fails to find a solution, when he or she is at a loss about what action to take, then the appropriate physical organ reacts as needed.

Four Shades of Biological Meaning

Illnesses play a biological role in survival. Each of them "adds" something helpful to a body in difficulty. For example, ulceration of the coronary arteries allows a better blood flow that can be enlisted in the body's ongoing struggle. A diabetic rise of blood sugar brings energy into the body's muscular system; a melanoma or a wart constitutes a protective shield; short-term memory loss allows the individual to avoid being confronted by anything that might reawaken the suffering brought on by a separation. This is the sense and significance of an illness.

Organs are logical assemblages of differentiated cells. Identical cells form tissue, and several tissues form an organ—a layer of muscle is combined with a mucous layer, for example. A conflict including several subtle aspects of a feeling can involve various tissues of the same region. Just as it is possible to classify biological conflicts into four basic families, it is also possible, for didactic purposes, to roughly classify the tissues that make up the physical bodies of living creatures into four large families of functions, and consequently, to find the four large families of biological meanings for the kinds of illnesses that affect them.

1. *Vital conflicts*. The operative metaphor here is "hiring extra help." The orchard or vineyard owner hires seasonal workers for the harvest, and factories sometimes hire temporary workers to meet an increase in demand.

   Biologically, the tissues affected by these conflicts form tumors, additional masses of cells that give the organ the ability to perform more work (an adenocarcinoma in the lungs to better oxygenate the blood, one in the liver to better extract and create reserves, one in the prostate to better adapt the sperm to the female genital tract to optimize the chance of procreation, and so forth).

2. *Conflicts of protection*. Here the metaphor concerns the role played by down in ensuring survival. During the warm months, horses have a layer of fine hair over their bodies, but in early winter they grow a thicker coat to protect them during the colder months ahead.

   The biological meaning of these kinds of illnesses is that the tissues involved also form tumors as an additional cell mass to provide a more effective kind of protection (melanomas, warts, cancers of the peritoneum and the pleura, and sun tanning).

3. *Self-depreciation conflicts*. The operative metaphor is the disappearance of windmills from most of our rural landscapes. With the introduction of electricity to rural areas, mills with electrical motors replaced the windmills that once dotted the countryside, as these electric mills offered their owners greater flexibility. Windmills therefore vanished fairly rapidly from the

rural landscape as they were gradually pulled down and their materials recycled. To maintain something perceived as serving no purpose is an impossible luxury.

Another illustration of this biological conflict is the pruning of branches. When a tree that grows next to a person's house has too many heavy branches, the homeowner may decide to manage the growth of the tree to keep its branches from falling on the roof of the house. The "branches" that are perceived as superfluous and useless in the brain of this individual are cut off or, in other words, pruned.

Biologically, the tissues affected by these conflicts (bone, muscle, conjunctive tissue, cartilage, discs, tendons, ligaments, and so on) lose substance and density. They disappear by completely or partially divesting themselves of their substance (osteoporosis, leukopenia, cartilage loss, thrombocytosis, shrinking muscles, atrophy) when an individual feels devalued in comparison to another person, or in a specific area, or in the person's ability to achieve a goal.

The brain then removes all or part of the organ that was designed by evolution to achieve its respective goal. To continue maintenance of an organ perceived as ineffective goes against nature. The organ or body part then starts receiving less fluid and food from the body and may even vanish completely.

Think of the osteoporosis of astronauts who, in space, are weightless. The reduction of the skeleton's usefulness (due to the almost total disappearance of certain mechanical tensions the bones are customarily under) triggers demineralization of the bones.

Another example: A woman devalues her own worth because she no longer has the manual dexterity necessary to embroider; another woman's parents have refused to give her hand in marriage to her intended. Both women will create a pathological condition of their fingers.

The clan forms a "living entity"—a cluster of individuals. Let an individual member of this cluster feel that he or she is underachieving, and all or part of the clan structure ceases to maintain that individual. The nutrients that are saved are virtually or actually put at the disposal of the clan.

4. *Conflicts based on relationships and territory.* The metaphor of choice here would be the dredging of rivers and canals. To allow more water to flow in riverbeds and ditches, humans dig and dredge deeper channels to enable the water to flow more quickly and in much greater volume.

Biologically, the tissues affected by territorial conflicts ulcerate and hollow out, thus allowing the volume of fluid that flows through them to increase. These illnesses shrink distances and durations, (stomach ulcers, bladder ulcers, cervix ulcers, for example). Breakdowns or disorders of the endocrine glands (insulin production, glucagon production, messenger molecules) organize substances that can be made available to either stimulate or inhibit an action.

Another metaphor is the stampede to ski areas and other vacation sites at certain times of year. On public holidays, when many people plan to take their vacations, the demand for transportation is such that railroad companies increase the numbers of cars headed for the resort destination, so that all vacationers can be sure of finding a seat. Meanwhile, in other parts of the country where there are no ski areas, there are fewer cars in circulation on the other trains.

Yet another metaphor is that of mountain guides and sherpas: When several things have gone astray in dramatic fashion, the astute mountain guide, realizing that these things can happen in a series, takes no chances on venturing into the mountains but waits for the situation to take a turn for the better.

The biological meaning of motor paralysis is that it leads to the restriction of movement or perception at a time when movement or perception could have tragic consequences. Multiple sclerosis puts a person on the sidelines and forces those around the person to move in his or her stead.

Now that we have established that illness arises in response to an intense emotion and not just at the whim of destiny, and that illness disappears following a hot phase, the reader should be able to understand that illness dissolves a mass of intolerable stress and brings assistance to an organ. The protective, guardian-angel side of illnesses should now be apparent. Illness is clearly a biological solution.

Illness Is Also an Invitation

Every spring, in cyclical fashion, green leaves push forth from the soil of the garden. Only then does the invisible tulip bulb reveal its existence and location. This extremely natural and constantly renewing phenomenon reminds us that perceptible visible matter is only the expression of the invisible (a memory, a plan) that precedes it. Through analogy, our symptoms invite us to become aware of their hidden causes.

All Illnesses Are Caused by Biological Conflicts

Here is an observation that is heard quite often: "Tendonitis in a tennis player is clearly caused by playing tennis; it is a mechanical problem, not a psychological one." The response to that is both yes and no. Not everyone who plays tennis develops tendonitis, so there must be a distinguishing element.

Tendonitis is due to a self-depreciation conflict created because a person is unable to immediately attain a goal that could have been attained with the involved limb. During a competitive tennis match, the player's conflict triggers the process leading to tendonitis. If the player can manage to play with a different state of mind, he or she will no longer create a pathological state centered on the tendon.

Here is another frequently heard remark: "Ever since I put my child in daycare (or in school), he has been sick constantly. It is clearly the fault of contagious germs." Again, the response is yes and no. If all the children experienced the same illness at the same time, it would mean they were resolving, or attempting to resolve, the same existential problem at the same moment.

Germs allow organs to perform a certain kind of repair, but they do not trigger illness. Generally speaking, a certain number of children remain healthy carriers and do not create an infection, or create it later if they haven't done so earlier. This is because the transition from home to daycare, with its setting of "common mothers" and "common activities," can trap at least some children who happen to be in the same transitional stage. At this period of life the child may experience separation conflicts, territorial conflicts—"That's *my* toy!"—as well as conflicts arising from problems of adequate self-expression, loss of contact with the mother, resentment, not having instant access to a parent, and so on. This makes a child very susceptible to the surrounding state of mind, and the child eventually tries to resolve the dilemma. When the child does resolve one or more of these conflicts, the child's brain triggers the hot phase of the reparation, which uses the germs that the daycare center makes available.

The classic childhood diseases are inevitable and accompany childhood development. They indicate that the child is managing to resolve conflicts (the grief of no longer being an only child, mourning the loss of the kind of contact with the mother the child once had, and so on) and is becoming more of an individual by isolating himself or herself from those things on the outside that were once felt to be a part of the child's own self.

The Common Cold

As the common cold is probably the most frequently occurring illness, it seems a worthy subject for further discussion here. The nose serves several purposes: letting in air, filtering, it, reheating it, carrying it to the olfactory cells, finding the spatial origin of an odor (for example, a baby finding its mother's nipple). The nose can also serve to analyze an environment from a distance, among other things.

The biological conflicts affecting the nasal mucous membrane have a relationship to these functions. As humans are naturally poorly armed (in comparison with lions, tigers, crocodiles, eagles, boa constrictors, and so on), surveillance plays more of a role in their survival than combat. The nasal mucous membrane conducts air to the olfactory cells. It regulates the volume of air and forms part of the individual's warning system, where to step next (who passed that way before one), what the sex of the individual approaching is, what kind of event may be about to transpire (one smells a fire, toxic gas, the presence of an animal, urine, wine, tobacco, and so on).

The wife and children of a chronic drinker use their noses to detect if the returning husband/father has been drinking and if so, how much, to know whether they need to protect themselves against any potentially aggressive behavior.

Some smells are pleasant because they are associated, for everyone, with memories of happy moments. Conversely, if an odor has been associated in the past with a highly stressful event (as the earlier section on allergies explained), this association can trigger the nose's automatic response to that stress.

Here is an equation that can serve as an example: Ether is used during an operation to remove a child's tonsils. During the operation, the child is alone, without parents, in the operating room, experiencing an invasive procedure. These factors create significant distress. Later, the slightest whiff of ether activates the anxiety connected to the memory of this event. The mucous membrane, which is on watch, then creates micro-ulcerations.

Because the archaic solution may be better informed of an imminent danger (the river reaching flood stage, a child who has not returned home from school, burglaries in the neighborhood, a man who is walking too close to another in the street, a bizarre or difficult relationship with a friend or lover), or when it is of vital necessity to "sniff out" an opportunity, to sense a "new wind" blowing in, a command may be given to the mucous membrane to make an ulcer. This enables a larger current of air to pass through the nose from which the olfactory cells can glean information. When the conflict has been resolved, rhinitis repairs the mucous membrane with the aid of viruses.

Human beings need a territory, a zone around them they can call their own. When this safety perimeter is reduced, they feel depression and alarm. Look at a packed elevator or an overcrowded bus to see how ill at ease people feel when they are forced to stand too closely together and social boundaries are violated. A feeling of intense unease, of which people are conscious to varying degrees, arises when the brain inventories its experiences that are associated with similar odors. Thus, the more frequently the source of the unease is experienced, the less chance the individual has of taking the unease into account. The individual will claim a virus picked up on the bus or in the elevator has caused the cold, although other people on that same bus will not catch the cold, either because they do not create that conflict or do so in a much less intense manner.

Psychiatric Illnesses

Humanity received another gift from Dr. Hamer; he revealed the etiology of *behavioral* disorders. Insanity is a particular cerebral state that is established when certain biological conflicts coexist.

A biological conflict presented to a cerebral stage, plus another conflict that develops at the same cerebral stage but affecting the other hemisphere, form a biological constellation that immediately triggers a mental disorder, rather than two physical illnesses. Although physical solutions to the conflicts are not solicited, the body is protected by the behavioral solution. (At one time, Freud supported the theory of cellular and physical origins of behavioral disorders, and we can make the observation today that his insight was on target.)

The simultaneous presence of two conflicts on the same cerebral stage is one too many. The individual is caught in a rotten past, and the assistance of two organs is not sufficiently adapted to the situation to enable the person to become free of it; outside actions are required, a new and bizarre kind of behavior by a super-persona, which can give the individual the ability to break from the past. He or she finds access to another dimension harboring a source of comfort and something extra, trump cards for resolving the problems.

Some examples: A conflict of resentment (gallbladder) and an identity conflict (rectum) form a constellation at the cortex, which necessitates violent behavior. The person this affects, whose calm and gentleness have been checkmated, may perhaps be able to resolve the problem by violence. A conflict of urgency and a conflict of head-on fear require lethargy and mystical delusion (which permits the individual to escape). A conflict of debasement and a conflict of the nest necessitate an emotional void (the absence of emotions, indifference) that allows the individual to act coldbloodedly and not be affected.

The discovery of this construct of biological constellations permits psychiatry to have its own revolution. Clinical observation and an examination of the patient's brain scans can indicate, among all these biological conflicts, which one—or more—should be resolved.

No one will be clinically insane or crazy for life any longer; madness will only last as long as certain biological conflicts are active.

My experience in treating a man by the name of Aldo is an example of this. Aldo had been released from prison, where he had been serving a sentence for assault with a deadly weapon (a knife). He had been compelled to get therapeutic treatment, and when someone from social services brought him to me, he was quite agitated and threatened to punch anyone who happened to accidentally bump into him in the street. The only information I had on him was the reason he had been imprisoned. The behavior of someone who uses a knife against others is steered by cerebral constellation of at least two simultaneously active biological conflicts, an identity conflict (left cortex) and a conflict of territorial resentment (right cortex).

In all probability, his brain would reveal these two focal points. Sitting down to talk with him over a few cups of coffee, I told him a story (invented) about a person who had lived a similar kind of a life, in which I emphasized *that* character's feelings of identity and resentment. This story hit the bull's eye, and Aldo, thus touched, became quite red, and developed both a fever and a brutal headache. In the space of a few seconds, he had swung to the other extreme, and he became polite and gentle. I saw him again two years later when he came to thank me. He had become a professional truck driver, and everything was going well for him.

In Conclusion

Humans have been expert in explaining the "how" of things for quite some time: the modalities of cancer, the relationship between the organs and the endocrine system, ion exchanges, membrane depolarizations, and so forth. But until the 1980s, we did not know how to respond to the question of why. Why cancer? Why (or, for what purpose) would one person develop rectal cancer and another cystic fibrosis? Illness is part of a consistent system permitting a super-homeostasis, the maintenance of an individual's life in an internal and external environment. It is the crutch that results from various pressures applied by reality, imagination, and symbolism to the human brain. Hence the necessity to evolve, grab onto a cure, and not backslide.

The four correlations between conflicts and illnesses presented in this text have been observed and verified dozens of times, even hundreds and thousands of times, for the most commonly occurring illnesses. The proof of their validity is provided by the presence of a cerebral focal point at the right spot, and especially by the cure of the patient, which begins the moment the conflict is resolved (or at the moment the emotional shock is consciously reexperienced).

Illness is a dangerous kiss from an angel.

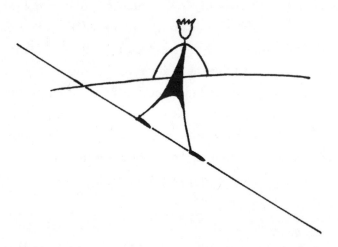

Figure 6.1. Illness is the balancing pole that allows people to reach the end of their journey.

SEVEN

CANCER EXPLAINED

Cancer is an illustration of the power of life.
PROFESSOR LUCIEN ISRAËL,
CLINICAL CANCER SPECIALIST

Cancer is a reflexive means of escaping the inevitable.
MARC FRÉCHET,
BIOLOGICAL DECODING PIONEER

A Tumor Always Serves a Useful Purpose

Cancers and tumors have long been perceived as anarchistic processes that act without any plan or meaning and follow only their own whims. This interpretation—for that is what it is—assumes that nature can experience moments of madness and display supernatural behavior. If humans have accepted this hypothesis, it is because it has allowed them to fight against cancer, rather than go along with it.

It was easier to divide life into two camps, one good and one evil, than to perceive the perfection of the world in everything. With eyes fixed firmly on the visible symptom rather than the invisible and fleeting feeling, humankind found reason to believe in the corruptibility of life, and thus came to believe itself naked and fragile. So humans stitched together some fig leaves, and this gave them some protection. And they died of fear.

Everything Is Adaptation

The body is in a constant quest for balance, just like the cyclist who implements thousands of solutions (muscular and nervous) to avoid falling, without always being aware of doing so.

The etymology of the word *symptom* gives us the word *coincidence*. A symptom, whether it is of cancer or something else, coincides perfectly with what the individual is experiencing. The order to make a cancer is always given by the brain to the cells involved by way of a very elaborate communication system. (This mind-gene communication is described in E. Rossi's book *Psychobiology of Mind-Body Healing*, New York: W. W. Norton, 1993.)

When game is plentiful, the lioness gives birth to several cubs. When it is scarce, she gives birth to only one, if any. This is adaptation. The human body adapts to every problematic circumstance. Tanning, for example, protects the body from an excess of solar radiation.

What does *benign* mean? Is tanning benign, or is absence of tanning benign? It's absurd to perceive a fundamental difference between a benign tumor and a malignant one. The devil of our religious mythology is the Adversary, who disturbs the established order and forces things to evolve. There is nothing benign or malignant involved, simply a progressive transition from normal cell to exceptional cell.

A cell that becomes cancerous is a cell that has taken courses in perfecting itself and in becoming more effective for the mission for which it is destined.

Intelligence, Not Anarchy

The particularly intense force of a biological conflict ensures that an organ produces what we call cancer. All the tumors of the cold phase, sprouting from identical tissues, look alike; they have the same form and the same organization. They vascularize and thereby become highly effective complementary organs that are able, depending on their nature, to secrete or absorb more. However, they always do this in the same way in all living things, plants and animals included.

This is the polar opposite of anarchy: it is operating in obedience to a plan.

If cancer were truly anarchic, a breast tumor in a Japanese woman would not resemble the breast tumor of an Englishwoman living on the other side of the globe. But not only does the cellular division, then multiplication, end up creating the same hard ball, but, in addition, an identical network of vessels sustains this "new" organ. It clearly involves an organization similar to that of the original organs. If we are seeking to characterize the phenomenon by analogy, anarchy is clearly ruled out.

A minor biological conflict stemming from the inability to get past some event, some filthy incident, experienced with a feeling of betrayal, for example, creates slightly different and slightly invasive intestinal tissue, whereas a major incident or long-lasting conflict creates much more invasive tissues in the intestinal cells. It is the intensity and duration of the conflict that determines the size of the cancer.

When the conflict is either resolved or suspended, these cancerous tissues stop growing. Those who have had cancers and been cured of them, naturally or with the aid of treatments, have been healed because their conflict was resolved beforehand, whether they realized this connection or not.

The Theory of Cancer's Dangerous Potential to Spread Is Why Cancer Is Considered Life-Threatening

Cancer specialists say, "Cancer would be of no account if it were not for its tendency to become widespread." To provide a seemingly plausible explanation for the fact that, quite often, other cancers appear in the wake of an initial cancer, the idea has been generally accepted, over all other imaginable hypotheses, that cancerous cells possess the capability of escaping from the original cancer and contaminating other organs of the body. However, no observer has ever established the actual existence of such contamination. Although the contamination theory was unfounded, it was readily adopted because of its plausibility. This hypothesis, which offers similarities with microbial contamination between individuals, or with superstition (in which the contagious nature of hexes and good-luck charms is well known), was easy to accept.

But the reality is quite simple. A person who is creating several biological conflicts more easily creates several cancers to resolve all his or her problems. The individual's brain appeals only to the organs that have the authority appropriate to resolve—archaically, of course—these conflicts. Each new cancer is a physical solution, a symbolic compensation of a new conflict. Often, the diagnosis of cancer (or any other allegedly incurable disease) itself provokes one or more additional biological conflicts.

Thanks to these new cancers that establish themselves at the time the terrible diagnosis is learned, the patient does not die at once from stress but survives. The patient is on life support. Some time later, especially because a person diagnosed with cancer is likely to be receiving regular treatments and examinations, including X-rays, these new cancers are detected. However, they are not the result of contamination by the original cancer. They are new answers to new conflicts.

Therefore, if on hearing the diagnosis of cancer, the individual's emotional reaction is "I am afraid of dying," one of the individual's lungs will make a cancer. If the feeling is "I feel overwhelmed and worthless," certain vertebrae decalcify and lose substance. If the individual's main feeling is "What will become of my children?" the left breast (of a right-handed woman) creates a cancer.

Metastases

Cloning can remind us that every cell of the body contains the genes for all the other parts of the body. Metastases would be tumors consisting of cells that have taken on a new identity and new skills (cells of bone become cells of the breast, for example) when necessary, just as a social planner or a plumber can, on the weekend, become a gardener, a cook, a mother, handle a lawnmower or a food processor, or wash a baby.

The complexity of an intensely felt emotion is responsible for either metastases or a secondary tumor. Metastasis is the perfect result of two shades of one conflict. Here are some examples of these relationships. If the feeling is "I need the support of my mother," bone cells (cells intended to provide support) turn into galactogenetic cells for symbolically giving milk (maternal affection) and calcium for the bone involved. If the feeling is "I need to hurry up and get on with my life," metastases would be found in the lungs; pulmonary cells (responsible for carrying vital oxygen) mutate and become thyroidal (to help symbolically in speeding up the desire to live before it is too late and death arrives).

As there is nothing haphazard in the body, most likely there is no internal and hazardous contagion by wandering cells. The proof for this is provided by the healing of metastasis after a good decodage.

The Proof Provided by Cerebral Imaging

Every organ that manufactures a cancer has a short-circuited cerebral relay. If one person has six different kinds of cancer, a brain scan taken at that time shows six short-circuited cerebral relays. Of 1,000 people all having these same six cancers in the same locations in the body, all 1,000 have the same short-circuits in their cerebral relays, as these relays are located in the same parts of the brain for all human beings. If it were true that cancerous cells migrated around the body in haphazard fashion, would it be possible to systematically find these short-circuits always in the same parts of the brain? The answer is no. The "spread" of the cancer is due to multiple fears and newly generated biological conflicts.

Just What Do People Die From?

If cancer is a survival mechanism, then why do people so often die from it? Cancer, like other illnesses, grants the individual extra time to live. It prevents the body from dying immediately at the time the conflict makes its appearance. The individual, therefore, has been lent a certain amount of time in which to resolve his or her biological conflict. If the individual fails to resolve the major conflict, or does so too late, the cancer will have grown to a very large size, and when the infectious repair stage begins—if it even gets the signal to begin—the repair work necessary for healing can prove insurmountable for the individual.

There is a point of no return that cannot be safely passed. As with almost everything on this planet, excess is lethal. Too much water, too much sun, too much food, and too much money can have harmful, even fatal effects. The same is true for too much cancer.

Generally speaking, though, it is not the cancer itself that causes death. Fear (often due to the negative thoughts this topic inspires) holds a great deal of the responsibility for the fact that cancer may end in death. The psychological factor plays a large role: a person who thinks that he or she has lost, that nothing can help, is in a state of abnegation. The patient is influenced by auto-suggestion and, awaiting his death, makes it a self-fulfilling prophecy. The power of thought is so strong that any aggravation of suffering, due to reparative edemas, pain, or a microbial infection—mistakenly perceived to be "bad" signs—is enough to trigger death. Exhaustion due to malnutrition and/or pain, unresolved conflicts and the conflicts created by the diagnosis, the alternation between the hot reparative phase and the cold phase, the pressure caused by cerebral edemas, and the difficulty in obtaining good assistance can all prove fatal.

The Fear of the Thing

Being haunted by the thought of a disease can facilitate its actual appearance. Whatever we imagine carries a heavy weight. The belief that one has an ailing liver (because two family members died of liver disease, for example) can contribute to the etiology of a liver disease. Why? The brain "knows" the identity of humans' true enemy: fear. For nature (and therefore for the biological brain, not the psychological brain), cancer, or any other illness, is a solution, not a problem.

The problem, conversely, is fear, which can have considerable neurological effects that may even bring the heart to a stop because of abnormal rhythms and an overdose of neuro-mediators. Consequently, to avoid death, the autonomic brain does everything in its power to eliminate this fear or reduce its intensity. What means does it have at its disposal to achieve this? It cannot thwart the information coming out of the psychological brain, to which it is a slave, and suppress this fear. The only thing it knows how to do is to act on a cellular level and give the command to reactivate a cancerous growth or trigger an illness.

Let's examine the fear of falling. We can easily walk along a beam lying flat on the ground. However, if we try to walk along a beam that has been placed above a certain height, we either stand petrified or fall off. This is because we have the idea that walking on an elevated beam is difficult and dangerous—that is our fear. Fear is born from the unknown, from ignorance, which then invites the individual to forge all manner of delusional and fantastic representations of his or her symptoms. Thus, the symptom or the illness is regarded as a consequence of heredity, stress, pollution, bad luck, or perhaps even a spell cast by an enemy.

Yet cancer, like all illness, exists in obedience to a conflict. It grows as long as the conflict is active, and it stops growing and hovers between stagnant and slight growth when the conflict has been suspended and/or has achieved balance. The illness disappears or fossilizes once the conflict has been resolved or surpassed (when the feeling that gave it birth is no longer experienced).

Realizing that cancer is a simple adaptation brought about by an intense feeling, which is under the constant control of the brain, and that the brain can stop its progression at any time and even expel it when it no longer serves a purpose, reduces the level of fear. The cancerous individual will then be headed in the direction of a cure.

EIGHT

FRIENDLY GERMS

We have tons of information about viruses, but we have not sought out the impalpable force that moves them.

J. P. ESCANDE AND C. ESCANDE, *Biologies*

Since the time that microbes (germs) were first discovered, they have been held responsible for the triggering of many illnesses and suspected as the cause of numerous deaths. But the microbe is not responsible for either; at most, it bears responsibility for the particular shape an illness may take.

Healthy Carriers

Analysis of a sample of the mucus from the throat of any one of us today will show evidence of various microbes, even though we are enjoying good health. For our entire life we are carriers of billions of germs, not all of which will cause infection.

In epidemics, the medical personnel brought in to provide care do not necessarily share the feelings of the stricken populace and thus do not manufacture the disease, although they are in contact with the microbe. Of 100 people who are exposed to a flu virus or another kind of virus, only 3 or 8 or 60 of them will come down with an infection. Contamination does not necessarily produce infection. So what is it that makes the difference? What makes a healthy carrier—someone, for example, who is sero-positive and enjoying good health—suddenly manufacture an infection, that is, the hot period of the whole process of the illness? Could this come about simply because of a failure of the immune system? This is what is commonly believed. But beyond this basic explanation, why is illness seen to be illogical, insane, malign, and harmful?

Once we examine the impact of a conflict (and the intense emotion that causes it) on the body, and keep this in mind when looking at how phenomena unfold, we come to realize that the immune system is never defective. It is what it needs to be; it does what it has to do when it must, adapting to both the inner land-scape (memories, feelings) and the outside reality. If the immune defenses are weak, it is due to the conflict. If they are too strong, it is also due to the conflict. The immune system is like a lieutenant that obeys and gives orders. It is the interface between the microbe troops and the commander in chief, which is the brain. The first trigger of an infection is the command given by the brain.

Of greater import in this regard is the soothing period that follows the resolution of a conflict. The biological conflict has been settled and is now ancient history. What is new is the perception that the microbes have "awakened" and are hard at work only on the earlier altered tissue, which had been summoned to the rescue by the brain to resolve the conflict. Microbes excel in the elimination of foreign bodies (a splinter, for example); the destruction of a tumor; and/or the reconstruction of tissue in a different manner (to cite only a few examples).

The Microbe–Multicellular Organism Combination

As complex multicellular organisms such as plants and animals came into existence, microbes faithfully accompanied these life forms over the course of what science calls evolution. They co-evolved. Plant life, animal life, and human life—all are impossible without microbes. Every area on the planet today houses micro-organisms that have adapted to the needs of the multicellular organisms living there, just as plants and insects have co-adapted, through shrewd mutations, to maximize pollenization potential.

Our bodies house ten times more germs than the cells of which they are composed. In essence, we *are* microbes. Microbes, just like cells, have four kinds of problem-based reactions, stemming from both ordinary and extraordinary events such as glaciations, temperature change, predation, volcanic eruptions, meteorite impact, solar radiations, chemical changes in the environment or the atmosphere, lightning bolts, and so forth. Therefore, they mutated and adapted the same way our cells did.

This is the reason some microbes play a supporting role to the cells responsible for taking care of the body's vital needs (for example, Koch bacilli in the stomach or the pulmonary alveoli). Microbes play a supporting role with the cells responsible for protecting the body (meningococcal bacteria and the meninges), others with the cells in charge of the body's structure for movement (streptococcus and connective tissue), and those concerned with the cells of "territory and relationship" issues (the herpesvirus and epidermoidic cells).

Microbes and cells act in complicity. Every living cell communicates with its environment. The cell (whether it is a pulmonary cell, skin cell, nerve cell, or one that makes up intestinal mucus) was originally constructed from a single-celled being (algae, bacteria), and it is quite obvious that it easily communicates with the microbe that most resembles it and lives near or inside it. In nature, birds of a feather flock together and act as one in a magnificent symbiosis.

Until quite recently, we believed that an infection was an illness of its own, and we sought to eliminate it by giving battle to the microbes and strengthening the immune system. But we were overlooking the brain's capacity for triggering illnesses, veritable symbolic corrections to the distresses that are felt. Microbes *in vivo* (in a living being) do not become virulent on their own initiative. The organ needing them invites them to multiply, as does the brain.

The Excellent Effect of Microbial Intervention

An organ can repair itself without the help of microbes, but it takes longer, with the result that the tumors engendered during the cold phase of an illness are not destroyed and eliminated. Instead, they remain physically present, encysted and calcified, and visible in X-rays, although they are inactive "fossils." In modern life, as it was in the wild, it is in the best interest of wounded or sick individuals to recover *all* their physical powers as quickly as possible in order to hunt, harvest, work, keep watch, and defend themselves. The "microbial part" of the individual, consisting of rapidly reproducing individual germs, can eliminate tumors, expel foreign bodies (with pus), and restore or improve the condition of an organ much more rapidly than the "cellular part."

Harmful Germs?

Microbes are adapted to an environment in the same way that complex plant life, animal life (such as parasites and acarids), and human life are adapted to a habitat and the germs it contains. An individual who visits a foreign land and becomes immersed in a different culture encounters germs to which his or her body and lineage are not habituated. If the individual is in a biological conflict upon arrival, or if he or she creates a conflict in the country they are visiting, (arising, for example, from a fear of the new country and its culture that is so very different), the individual goes into a vagotonic state. The body will react at a high speed thanks to the new germs, and the speed of the repair can create a danger.

With an infection, it is the edema accompanying the repair of the cerebral relays that seems to pose a problem, not the microbial activity. *This is a distinction that we have not made before: Any repair of a part of the body is accompanied by the repair of its corresponding cerebral relay.* The higher the level of performance of the microbe in repairing the organ, the more rapid the speed of that repair. The more rapid the repair of an organ, the greater the cerebral edema, and the greater the danger it represents. Fortunately, cerebral edema can be reduced with sympathicomimetics (such as antibiotics, cortisone) and substances (such as aspirin) capable of pumping out the fluid accompanying edemas. In the past, results were obtained using such remedies without a clear idea of what was transpiring. The discovery of edema of the cerebral relay, edema that is concomitant and in proportion to the physical repair and microbial activity, provided us with the explanation we were lacking.

Any new germ an individual encounters is potentially hyper-effective. It requires several generations, or at least long adaptational periods, for an individual to reduce his or her sensitivity to this microbe. Consequently, a germ introduced as a weapon of war, for example, would be potentially fatal for only those individuals manufacturing a conflict corresponding to the tissue that is "cousin" to that germ. As the biological conflict that causes lung illnesses is the fear of death, it is easy to see how the simple threat of germ warfare can transform a healthy carrier of these germs into someone suffering from a serious lung ailment.

We should not lose sight of the fact that whatever germs one may carry or pick up, the *fear* of being contaminated by dangerous germs causes more disorders than the germ itself, as the brain reacts (with an illness) to lower that fear to a more tolerable level.

Pasteurization

Although the discovery of the germ by Pasteur and his team was obviously very significant, it was incomplete: They based their theories on microbial behavior *in vitro*, in the test tube (behavior that reveals little of import, as a germ behaves differently depending on whether the cellular tissue in which it lives is connected to a brain or not) and on microbial behavior *in vivo*, in a living being (which is equally valueless if consideration is not given to the conflicts of individuals and the feelings they experience).

In any event, vaccination became quickly accepted because it often seemed highly effective. However, this only *appeared* to be the case, as vaccinations were generally given when epidemics were in the process of disappearing naturally. The placebo effect produced by a vaccination campaign is equally relevant to this process.

Pasteur's theories were quickly accepted, and those who objected to his findings were soon forgotten. The world became accustomed to the equation: germs produce illness, while scorning the other equation: illness summons germs. Vaccine manufacturers have even recently succeeded in imposing their will on politicians (using fallacious arguments and inflated figures) with the campaign of incitement they have organized to compel inoculations against hepatitis B.

What has emerged is that, by rendering a microbe or virus harmless (with vaccination, for example), one specific type of illness becomes rare and disappears. This is in no way a victory against illness but against only one specific form of illness, because the body, once there is a conflict, adapts, modifies, and repairs itself. Other forms of disease then emerge that are just as troubling (the general disappearance of polio was accompanied by the more frequent appearance of various neurological scleroses), for the brain knows what germs it has at its disposal. Every family of microbes brings into the host body memories of specific distresses that interfere with the emotions and, therefore, with the behavior of the tissue of that body. Might not mandatory vaccinations bring about a certain kind of emotional uniformity in people?

The discovery of microbes also helped solidify the pattern of thinking in which the rational and demonstrable were given preference over the subjective and impulsive. For hundreds of years, before the discovery of microbes, when an illness or epidemic appeared in a village, witches (marginal members of the community) or strangers would be held responsible for the misfortune and were either exiled or murdered for their malefic actions, without the need for any kind of trial. After the discovery of microbes, the person who brought in the foreign germ would be quarantined and, in the best case, cured.

But today, with the quarantining of those contaminated by the corona virus, or the humiliation and isolation experienced by those who are HIV-positive, we can see that being labeled a carrier of germs (which causes fear) can still lead to death through the induction of biological fears and the conviction that the germs will cause one's death.

Today, however, a new threshold has been crossed, because, by clearing germs of the culpability too long associated with them, we have come to appreciate the excellence of nature. Everything is symbiotic, logical, adequate, and as harmonious in the depths of organisms as it is in the immensity of the universe.

An Indian proverb says: "The same spring cannot be both freshwater and saltwater." Likewise, how would it be possible for microbes to be indispensably useful in the digestive tract and harmful everywhere else?

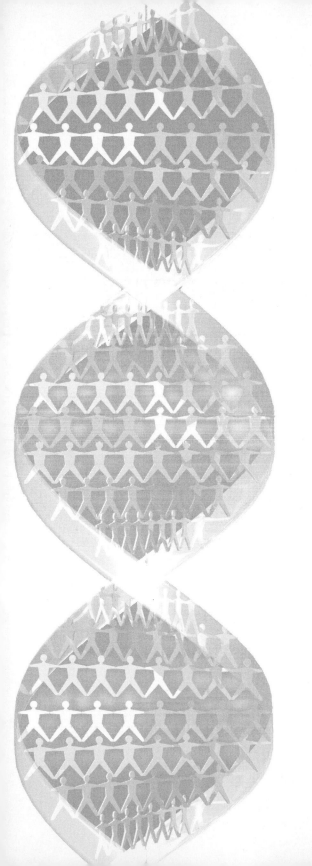

PART TWO
DESTINY

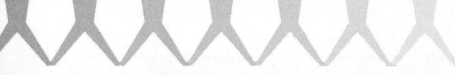

NINE

THE WHIMS OF DESTINY

When you criticize others for their failings, realize that the only failings you can see in them are your own.

Thanks to a row of plane trees planted on each side of the road, I was protected from the sun as my car was approaching Nice. I arrived there without mishap. I did not steer my car into one of these trees, despite their close proximity to the road. It was not my time to die.

However, many people have crashed their cars into these plane trees, as the bundles of flowers placed at various sites along the road testify. Yet despite the fact that all these drivers wanted to get safely to their destinations, something inside them took over the steering of their vehicles and prompted that second of inattention required to achieve a fatal collision.

The necessary and unknown chain of events known as destiny is easily perceived and invoked when our desires and ambitions prove impossible to satisfy, when the course of things seems more powerful than our consciously expressed choices. The swimmer who seeks to make it to the bank of the river and is prevented by the current quickly realizes that a more dominant force—the speed and direction of the water—is carrying him or her somewhere else. *Mekhtub:* "It is written."

This destiny that guides the lives of us all unfortunately does not have to take our desires into account, as it has other priorities. The origin of destiny, of fate, like that of illness, goes back to the dawn of time.

Destiny would be a chain that obliges the individual to go in a certain direction, to experience a certain situation. Why? Why did Jeanne get married when she was twenty-one years and nine months old? And why did her daughter Juliette get married at exactly the same age? Why did Joseph miss his flight on an airplane that subsequently crashed? Why did Elizabeth manufacture an intestinal tumor when she was thirty-four? Why did Rosa die at the age of thirty-nine from a thrombosis, whereas her grandfather Rudolph died at the same age when he was crushed by a falling tree?

What happened to make Gaston abandon his medical studies and emigrate to Argentina to raise cows? Why did Guy become ill just at the moment he became successful doing something he loved, and why did Andrew grow rich doing something that bored him to death? Why didn't Aline ever marry? Why is Patrick in permanent conflict with his father? Why did Vivian develop a pancreatic cyst, whereas her mother was dispossessed and cheated of her inheritance? Why do so many people exhaust themselves working and find, when all is said and done, that they are never justly compensated for their efforts? Was it because they chose this? No, they were guided to do so.

This remote guidance makes it possible to attain an objective whose hidden meaning escapes ordinary perception. But its hidden meaning cannot escape a targeted, intentional search. Is it necessary to accept a destiny that is so obviously unfavorable? Where the fatalist would say "Yes," the curious individual who seeks to evolve will answer "No."

So how are we to get out of a current that, in obedience to some logic, is carrying us in a direction we do not wish to go? By fighting it? No, for this struggle is often lost in advance, just like the one against illness. An anti-destiny is still a destiny. Taking advantage of the current is the more sensible course. The swimmer carried away by the river current, rather than fighting it and becoming exhausted by swimming against it, can exploit the current (by learning to understand it) and take a trajectory that proves more satisfactory.

Comprehension is liberating. By discovering the meaning of our destiny, we can learn to value it, to find serenity, to "win free will," to satisfy our yet-unsatisfied needs, just as through understanding the meaning of our illnesses we can heal ourselves.

Knowing why I have such a tragic destiny is already soothing and gives meaning to my misfortune; and, with the energy this knowledge gives me, I can, at the end of a sort of targeted search, give up my faithfulness to my family tree and trace out a road to abundance.

The earlier chapters have shown that illnesses have a meaning concerning survival inside of destiny. We are now going to look at how our behavior, our lifestyles, what we do and what we manage not to do, also have a meaning for our survival and the survival of our lineage.

Did You Say "Karma"?

Of Eastern origin, the word *karma* symbolizes the law of cause and effect. For example: I press on the brake pedal, and karmic law ensures that my car comes to a stop, that the car behind me passes around me, that a dead leaf is moved by the car going around me, and so on. The exploration of the different kinds of programming in the pages to follow clearly shows evidence of this law of cause and effect, but it is enriched with the notion of the meaning for survival that illnesses and destiny possess.

However, I will not use the word *karma,* as, in the West, it has taken on an inexact meaning of punishment or immutable influence, which adulterates its primary meaning. But everything is karmic, from the glass I break when doing the dishes, to the speed and shape of the cloud that is passing above you now.

Did You Say "Incarnation"?

The embodiment of a soul in a new body bears a strong resemblance to the installation of a software program on a computer. Everyone knows that a computer is useless without software, without the basic programming that permits it to perform. There is no such thing as a useful container without content. It is the program that this assemblage welcomes and supports, and that gives it a meaning. The living creature is also something more than a simple conglomerate of differentiated cells; it takes on a mission that gives it meaning. This is the biological meaning of its life.

The Larousse Dictionary defines "soul" as follows: "That which inside us thinks, feels, and desires." It is also "a small piece of wood that communicates vibration through every piece of a stringed instrument." [The French word for soul, *âme,* also means "sound post."] Imagine that this instrument is the individual's family tree, and that the parts of this tree are all the members of the person's family, both the living and the dead. The vibration would then be the lived history (including all the difficulties encountered by the person's ancestors). The soul, this small piece of wood, transmits this vibration to one's descendants. Communication is made necessary by an innate desire (one that is different from and complementary to conscious desire) to prepare the individual's progeny for the difficulties they are likely to meet.

This soul therefore consists of memories and souvenirs that

essentially arise from the lives of our ancestors and those close to them (those who resonate with them). The incarnation of the soul is a transfer of memories into the child, a transfer that takes place around conception. Of course, there are many other conventional definitions for the word *soul,* but in this book, the meaning I have just provided is the one that is pertinent.

The Phenomenon of Destiny and History

The notion of destiny, or fate, is found in every civilization, whether in its religions, its tragedies, or its foundational myths. Marc Fréchet reminds us that the Romans depicted destiny under the features of Fatum and Fortuna. The Greeks had the Moirae, a trio consisting of Clotho, Lachesis, and Atropos. Seated upon dazzling thrones of light, the youngest, Clotho, turned the distaff. Lachesis turned the spindle and the thread of the life of an individual, and Atropos, without batting an eyelash, cut the thread, thus irrevocably determining the moment of death.

Whether in Greek or Roman culture, destiny is a complex idea in which inflexibility, inevitability, chance, arbitrariness, whims, injustices, and favors are always present. The Greeks also observed that destiny, to which everyone is customarily bound, could have its course changed thanks to Tyche, another goddess. Tyche symbolized the complementary force that can be translated as the impact of our awareness of what is guiding us.

The realization of the origin of a destiny can enable us to change our trajectory from a current that makes sense for our lineage, our branch, but not necessarily for us on an individual level. Free will asks for the proper "touch," the proper connection with a moment contained within the family distaff.

The deterministic nature of destiny is very good at alleviating guilt, whereas the postulate that we can choose between "good" behavior and "bad" behavior is politically much more potent, as it involves controlling a populace and making people docile. It can easily be seen why astrology—once a science taught to priests and astronomers, which reveals the hyperdeterminism that governs the lives of humans—was banned in the fourteenth century by the Church of Rome.

The Law of the Clan, or Phylocentrism

Our behaviors and all the paths we take throughout our lives may be considered to be "primitive" solutions to the unresolved problems of our infancy, our birth, our intrauterine life, and of several generations of our family trees—our earlier lives, in fact.

Warning: We cannot understand destiny and adjust our destiny if we perceive ourselves as separate, as "individual individuals," from the trunk of our family tree. That is because a lineage—in other words, us combined with our ancestors—is like a vine snaking through the forest canopy and drawn upward by the nourishing sunlight. This lineage is greedy for the future, for what is yet to come. The transmission of life from one individual to the next is like a game of leapfrog that connects us to our most remote ancestor who has passed on to us a single cell living in the primordial sea of life.

Because time is quite old and is always extended toward the future, it has no meaning, and the needs of the lineage are not the same as those of the individual. The individual, one link in the chain of the family line, wishes to have a house and a comfortable car, more than enough money, a flourishing sex life, healthy children, friends, recognition for accomplishments, and so on. But our personal desires, no matter how legitimate they appear to be to us, are not priorities. Try to grasp the extent of this egocentrism to get a better idea of the invisible reality of what I call "phylocentrism." Phylocentrism sums up the fact that our life is subordinate to and subjugated to our lineage *(phyla)* and its purpose: eternal life. It is therefore the opposite of egocentrism, in which everything is brought down to the level of the ego, to the individual. Paradoxically, though, forging a connection to this phylocentric reality enables us to perhaps later satisfy our basic, egocentric desires for love, contact, and other essential needs.

Did You Say "Choice"?

At certain times in our lives, we think we are choosing the direction we will be going. However, we often choose nothing, not where we live, nor our frequent associations, nor our professions. Our profession, for instance, is, like the choice of an illness, the means by which we often seek to protect ourselves from some old, resonant, hidden pain.

Becoming an interior decorator is the solution to a conflict based on an aesthetic self-depreciation. Spelunking may be the solution to a conflict connected with a mother (in the family tree) who may not be one's real mother (returning to Mother Earth in search of verification). As long as we remain completely ignorant of certain dramatic past experiences, we spend our lives revolving around them and reproducing them, in order to reveal them. And while this is taking place, our legitimate desires are defied. As long as we are ignorant of them, we are nothing but the loyal and obedient leaves of an old tree.

To be an "individual" individual requires effort and a kind of initiatory approach. The first efforts require discernment: How do I detach myself from these missions if I cannot even see or feel the strings, the threads (in other words, my automatic loyalties) that go from the marionette that I am to the trunk of the tree that manipulates me? Where do I need to cut these familial strings to gain my freedom and satisfy my *own* personal needs?

Let's assume, for the sake of argument, that a father in the lineage may not have been one's biological father, and that this fact was kept hidden. One or more descendants may have their lives

98

driven in such a way as to bring this fact to light. Two conflicting, opposite behaviors work to reveal the secret.

One descendant will either be strong in algebra and history, or have absolutely no talent for these two subjects. These two opposing behaviors are actually two ways of reacting to the same secret connected to one's ancestral line of descent. Excelling at history (much of which is a narrative chronicling the lineages of kings) and algebra (the search for X, the unknown) on the plus side denotes a curious and aggressive nature (to pierce the secret) in a child, whereas having no talents in either of these subjects reveals the child's essentially passive nature. Later, when the child has reached adulthood, he or she will seek out a similar situation. This person may have a child whose existence is concealed, or the theme of the secret child or the illegitimate father may enter into the person's life in some other way.

Johanna had been raped repeatedly from the time she was sixteen until she was eighteen, by her boss and one of his friends. She was so ashamed of having been the consenting victim for such a long period that she could never admit to anyone what had transpired. Later in life, Johanna had a son who was alarmed at his fascination with photos of naked men. This fascination, whose meaning eluded him, caused him great anxiety and guilt. The excessive stress of his mother, colored by disgust and transgression (sex is a sin), lack of respect (due to the rape), and guilt (because of whatever pleasure it had given her nonetheless), was obviously associated with men in one of these equations that the brain is so skilled at establishing, memorizing, and passing down to one's descendants.

The woman's unrevealed situation, which had been kept secret because it was inadmissible, was automatically passed on to her son. The fascination he experienced was simply due to the fact that he had inherited a kind of overstress that was unidentified and undated, and he was seeking to rid himself of it through his compulsive behavior.

The unspoken, ingrained suffering of his mother (colored by the guilt connected to the presence of men with erections) could not be eliminated, and thus the son was steered to a highly symbolic, similar form of behavior.

The analogical nature of one of the brain's functions makes it so that the suffering of a victim also leaves its mark on the unconscious of the victimizer. The soldier on campaign who rapes women, once he has returned home, will guard his silence about his criminal acts and therefore inject into his future children a certain number of equations and hidden emotions that can haunt his descendants for generations. How often have the paths of the descendants of victims and those of their torturers crossed without their knowing it?

As Carl Jung said, "Everything that has not been revealed expresses itself in the form of fate."

Here is another poem to illustrate the points made in our chapter.

Good Morning USA

A swimming champion
was expected to win a gold medal
at the Olympic Games.
She was faster than all her rivals.
The day of the games, something amazing occurred.
When she was leading the pack at the beginning
of the last length of the pool,
she practically stopped swimming, just enough to allow
the woman who was behind her, an American swimmer
to carry away the Gold Medal.
She later learned
that her grandmother
who she hardly knew
practically worshipped Americans

because they saved her family.
Her cousin had even successfully
played a role in the expansion of
a well-known American company!
But this champion had been unaware
of all this before the Olympic games.
Then, when the time came,
homage was paid to the American nation.

The Personality

Personality is what characterizes us, both in the eyes of others, and to ourselves. It then evolves at the will of our professional and emotional conflicts that tip us over in accordance with precise biological rules, from a feminine form of behavior to a masculine one, and vice versa: One moment I am buried in my work, at another moment I want to be with my children and not work at all.

A macho or an extreme feminine attitude, tomboyishness in a woman or effeminacy in a man, are the consequences of the impact of conflicts on the brain. The personality of an individual can thus be considered to be a result of what he or she felt at birth and during the formative years, and it is with this personality that the individual carries out what has been programmed for his or her entire life. The education that one receives, with its taboos and parental or collective neuroses, will interfere in the destiny of one's descendants.

The Moment of Death

What are the means human beings use to die, to seal off the time-space to which an individual has been responsible for giving life, after having passed on the baton in a relay to the following generation, in a corridor of time on the great terrestrial stage? All peoples have their own ways of dying. The fact is that one must clearly die of something, and while it is true that death occurs only when the heart stops, it is still necessary for the programmed body to have a "lever" that causes the heart to stop. A conflict that endures for far too long, an overly rapid onset of vagotony, a blow to the integrity of the circulatory system, poisoning, not enough food, suicide—these are all levers at the service of the different varieties of programming.

The African child uses the amoeba from standing water to bring about the time of death set by his programming; the driver employs a tree or a tractor-trailer; the cautious person uses conflicts and beliefs to make a cancer fatal.

While the time of death can sometimes, thanks to an observation made *a posteriori,* correspond to someone else's that preceded it—a deceased ancestor who died at the same age or on the same date, for example—it is abnormal for children to die before their parents. It is against both logic and nature to die after one's children. To die before one's time is programmed when an ancestor or ancestors experienced excessive stress at a certain age. A descendant may escape this stress by dying just before its onset, but this premature death represents a waste of energy for the lineage. In the plant kingdom, when a plant, a branch, a leaf, or a fruit dies before attaining its normal development, basic survival mechanisms ensure that other parts of the plant reestablish the inner homeostasis with new sprouts in compensation.

Likewise, when an individual dies prematurely, the task of taking care of the unresolved conflicts of the lineage is reapportioned among the living and among those yet to be born.

TEN

THE DESTINY OF CHILDREN IS THE GUARANTEE OF THE SPECIES' SURVIVAL

The tree is a three-dimensional space
In which the past is always present.
In the treehouses of our youth
We are looking for our past, greedy for the future.

The paths we take in life, with our tastes, penchants, and physical or mental illnesses, are all perfectly logical solutions to the problems of ancient generations.

An Hour That Weighs Heavily

When an hour (or a minute) has been experienced in a profoundly weighty fashion (one that is dangerous, emotionally painful, or clashing, or which presents an apparently insoluble problem), that hour (which is also a geographical position in space in the earth's orbit around the sun, a specific location that is defined by established reference points) is underscored, in the souvenir album inherited by new generations from the old, as representing a danger. Therefore, succeeding generations carry, within that family's epigenetic information, the fact that that particular hour is dangerous and, when the earth places a descendant in this same sidereal position, or when any kind of stimulus indicates this hour, the feeling of the former clash manifests itself (such as an anniversary, for instance). The descendant responds with an action (a destiny, a choice, a behavior, or an illness). Of course, this hour may be only a minute, it may be a second, or even several weeks. This is the principle that governs allergies. The allergen is therefore a precise moment of the year. Some people feel poorly at a given time of the year, although this moment does not signify anything particularly difficult or painful for them.

Sacrifice

It would not be erroneous to think that creating a cancer, living a life of misery, or having a successful career in business, simply to compensate for the inadequacy of an ancestor or to resolve a problem, falls under the heading of sacrifice. This "sacrificial" form of functioning is actually widespread in nature. We can also find this kind of interdependence and sense of sacrifice in matter itself.

For example, if we take a sheet of metal or cardboard and subject it to an "unexpected" pressure—one that takes it by "surprise," as it were—it adapts and preserves this adaptation in memory in the form of a crease or a fold. If subjected to pressure a second time, the sheet folds more easily in the same place it did the first time. Thanks to this facilitation, the rest of the sheet is kept safe. This is how nature limits breakage. The different parts are interdependent to ensure the survival of the whole. Individuals count for little in this regard; their lineage is everything. Of what use is a small fragment of cardboard? Only the sheet itself is useful.

The family is also a molecule, composed of atoms that are invisibly linked to one another. Multicellular organisms such as human beings, who appear to be physically autonomous and free to wander as they will across the surface of Spaceship Earth, are in fact permanently connected to their genealogical tree. We are not as autonomous as we might believe, because the information that we have taken in unknowingly guides us with clockwork precision.

Becoming Informed Is Always the Best Way to Adapt

The winning solution that ensures the perpetuation of the life of the line consists of alerting generations to come about the difficulties encountered by their ancestors. Through the ties of blood (memory of water, epigenetic organization, etc.) children receive a family souvenir album rich in information with regard to all the dangers that have been met in the past. The future is always built on the foundations of the past. When a house has been destroyed by a tornado or flood, its inhabitants invariably rebuild it differently or in a different spot, because they carry in mind the memory of what happened. Similarly, progeny are conceived with a specific relationship to something in the past, and in accordance with what it was that took place.

Every excessive distress that cannot be successfully dealt with by an individual through thought or deed—a stress that has exceeded the tolerance of that person's psychological brain—goes into the blood, where it may lie dormant for a long time. From the mother's blood to that of the baby, from one brain to the next, this information is passed down in a steady stream.

An excessive stress dating from 1897 can be read one day by the brain of a descendant in 1957. A child may be born with one or more organs that are more effective (bigger or smaller, or better adapted) than those in the bodies of either of the parents. Sometimes the genetic information passed down comes with even greater force from the family trees of *both* parents, and the child is born with an atypical organ that doctors label as "diseased"— a congenital incapacitating disease, for example. Or the child may be gifted with a special talent instead.

Morphological innovations (a larger nose, or the heart on the right side of the body, for example) and congenital diseases (such as muscular dystrophy, spina bifida, cleft spine, cystic fibrosis, or Down syndrome) are examples of biological responses that are adaptations to the problems experienced by earlier generations.

The progeny, throughout the cosmic journey that is its life, lives through numerous different experiences, but has a strong reaction to only *some* of these experiences. For an individual to be concerned by a particular event, his or her souvenir album must already include memories of excessive distress corresponding to this same kind of event. The descendant then relives the past of the family tree.

The first half of this book touched on the two kinds of solutions that the brain can adopt. One involves the cell, which changes its own behavior inside the body (illness is a physical solution). The second consists of sending the individual into another dimension, the "Hamerian Constellation" (depression, madness, psychosis, phobias, and so forth), a solution that is both physical and behavioral.

But there is a third solution. The individual can be unconsciously compelled to adopt either a lifestyle, an activity, a kind of behavior, a profession, or a place to live (as a symbolically reparative environment), to take different directions in life that are in fact relational solutions of the body inside its surroundings. If the problem is something that can be resolved by a particular lifestyle, a specific job, a certain hobby, or meeting this or that person, then the organ is no longer on the front lines taking the brunt of the distress, and the *entire life* of the individual becomes the biological solution.

When seawater becomes less transparent, the descendants of the algae living there either go live somewhere else—that is, to a place where there is more light—or modify some of their cells to improve their output, so that the diminished amount of solar energy is sufficient to meet their needs.

When there is a reduction in the amount of oxygen in the water, the fish that can no longer adapt expedites this distress into its gametes, so that its descendants are born with more powerful gills or with the message to seek a new place to live.

When a person experiences distress because he or she cannot mark off territory and thus keep it, and if the person is unsuccessful at resolving this problem, then either the person or one of his or her descendants will adopt, without knowing why, a symbolically compensatory profession (customs agent, fencing salesman, arms merchant, alarm inventor, night watchman, and so on), or the person or the descendants might have the kidneys manufacture kidney stones (the urinary lithiasis furnishes the individual with the stones needed to construct a "stone" wall). Strong-smelling urine is the optimum physical solution for this conflict, as it symbolically enables the individual to mark territory, just as animals do.

A couple who owned a large property (where the entire family often gathered, and which was the pride of the clan) were victims of blackmail and forced to sell this property for peanuts. Thirty years later, one of their grandsons, who was experiencing a territorial conflict provoked by the daily invasion of his office by his boss, manufactured numerous episodes of nephritic colic and periods of depression.

It Takes Two to Make One

Sexual reproduction was adopted by nature concomitantly with asexual reproduction because it permitted rapid evolution of the species through successive mutations—an evolution crucial to the survival of the species.

But sexual reproduction and the abandonment of schizogenesis brought with it the death of the individual, which would occur at the end of a life's journey of varied duration. The child arrives to replace the elder; this is how birth is connected to death. The bamboo flowers but once, then dies, just like the grasses growing along the side of the road when their time is up.

There is an old saying that expresses this scenario well: "A birth pushes a death, a death pushes a birth." When a child is born, the event is quite often accompanied by the death of an ancestor or close relative that same year. The child then receives some of its programming from that individual. While the individual will one day return to dust, the information received at birth—enriched, purified, and transmitted to his or her descendants—continues to live on.

Before fertilization, the phenomenon of cell division (meiosis) among the reproductive cells provokes, in a clever manner, the loss of half the chromosomes. The egg creates a receptacle to house the memories of the spermatozoon, and the spermatozoon reciprocates. The progeny is conceived by two historically and biologically compatible souvenir albums, which set up a shared resonance based on what they have in common. A transfer of the parents' information to the egg is made outside the awareness of the parties involved.

This kind of transfer is the most reliable method in existence; none of the bad experiences and problems that have hitherto gone unsolved run the risk of being forgotten. Everything can be forgotten but that which has been deeply buried, frozen in time, and engraved on cells (water-memory, epigenetic organisation, proteins, etc., for the more recent memories) and on the DNA (for the most archaic pieces of information). It is impossible to disobey orders that one is not aware of having received. The child is the keeper of the souvenir album that he or she will be able to read only through the interface of the child's own life and actions.

The Drawbacks of the Programming

The ancestors have bequeathed to their children the memories of problems they were incapable of resolving, telling them, "I am alerting you to what happened to me so you can take your own steps accordingly." This system for the transmission of dramatic memories seems to have been valued more highly in earlier times than it is today, times when individual lifespans were, on average, much shorter than they are now. The new individual arrived several minutes or several hours after conception into the great cosmic ferment and found itself confronted at once by a problem, the very same problem encountered by its mother and father, its grandparents and great-grandparents. Therefore, adaptation via the mutation of some of its cells was immediately useful, enabling it to live.

But the lifespan of living organisms grew longer and longer. Between the moment in which a being, over-distressed by a dramatic event that had no solution, enriched its souvenir album with this information (or projected it into the family unconscious, from brain to brain until the descendant made it their own), and the moment when a child is born and begins growing, a certain amount of time elapses, several months or even several years.

Over time, that problematic situation (of the father, the aunt, or the grandmother) may have disappeared. However, the descendant is born armed to confront that scenario that no longer exists. (An underdeveloped ear auricle, for instance, could be designed to prevent one from hearing an intolerable noise or word; or a case of muscular dystrophy would prevent one from performing an inappropriate gesture or movement, and so on.) The descendant's hearing difficulty or lack of an ear auricle, or his or her muscular dystrophy, have actually become handicaps.

These programming packages make our individual natures distinctive; each of us is unique. They are delivered to us secretly, and the information (the date, the place, the circumstances, the "feeling" of the first overstress, or that of an ancestor's) that could inform us about the obsolescence of a problem is not delivered clearly either. The spatiotemporal data of the initial problem are present, though; and the body knows where this different programming comes from. It is up to us to make the body speak so we can find healing. Hence the advantage of decoding these illnesses, destinies, and behaviors with people who are trained therapist-decoders.

To free yourself from the obligations these problems present, it is necessary to direct your conscious mind to what some of your ancestors lived through. If this is not done, the automatic pilot remains fully operational for want of awareness, for lack of light, and destiny unfolds inexorably to its predetermined conclusion, whether it is the destiny of a cell or the destiny of an individual.

This mechanism of transgenerational transmission seems so primary and so archaic that we might think modern humans evolved past it long ago. But human beings continue to evolve, and the system is still in play. Illnesses and destiny are balancing poles that allow individuals and their lineages to walk along the tightrope overlooking the great cosmic void without falling, even if the balancing pole sometimes seems a bit too heavy to carry.

ELEVEN

THE PROGRAMMING

The Main Kinds of Programming for Living Creatures

Each of us is the result of millions of biological conflicts that have been experienced and deeply felt during millions of years of evolution. The most recent of these conflicts form the different programs of our destiny.

These different kinds of programming can be divided into four categories.

Archaic coding. This concerns the ancient history of the various lineages, with the species framework that ensures all the individuals of the same species display common characteristics. Ducks have wings, fish have scales, Africans are black, differentiated cells are able to mutate, African women have shorter menstrual cycles than Swedish women, and so forth.

Transgenerational programming. The unresolved problems of the ancestors ask the following generations to find solutions. "Souvenir albums" are handed down from one generation to the next for this purpose.

Unknowing parental projection (or projected meaning). This concerns what the parents experienced and felt deeply around the time of conception, during gestation, and after the birth of their child.

Before and during conception, the events that caused significant conflicts for the parents are analogically imprinted into the child. In what ambience is the child conceived, for whom, and why? What member of the family died during this same period? Was the person born during an economically flush time for the parents, or during a period characterized by failure, separation, and illness?

What exact programming was created by what the embryo experienced *in utero*? What did the mother feel during gestation? What new equations were established by the new being's presence? Is the child the fruit of a joyful and vibrant coupling from an ecstatic moment shared by the mother and father, or was it conceived without shared pleasure and for the mere reason that when people marry, they are supposed to have children? What happened to the parents during the nine months of the mother's pregnancy? Did the family move during this time? Were there any radical changes in their lives?

Then, after the child was born, what happened to it during the first months of infancy? What were the first trials of that child's life: finding one's mother's smell again; obtaining food, attention, love, and protection. What were the different excessive distresses (the arrival of another child, the death of a parent or relative) that the child experienced during the oral stage (birth to eighteen months) or during the anal stage (eighteen months to three years)?

Childhood experience. This includes the stress experienced during the phallic ("Oedipal") stage, and the nature of the relationship between the child and the parents. The relationship between the child and its brothers and sisters also necessitates later behavioral reactions and reverberations.

Only the constructs of transgenerational programming and

unknowing parental projection are fully explored here, as they form the skeletal structure of how the individual will use his or her time in the future. There are many specialist works that deal with the other kinds of programming.

Does Time Exist?

The minute one begins talking about programming and programs, time becomes a factor, either exact times—such as Friday, September 8, at 10:00 in the morning—or cycles of varying duration, such as a period of ten years, or of five years, four months, and thirteen days.

The existence of the phenomenon of trangenerational programmings leads us to reconsider our notion of time. Given the phenomenon of transgenerational programming, couldn't time be considered to be a human illusion? It would seem that it has little importance for our biological reality and cellular memories. Consequently, if this were the case, would space then have a greater reality?

Our habit of dividing the day into hours and the year into seasons and months helps us overlook the fact that at every instant we are occupying a very precise position in the universe. The date of birth, the wedding date, or the time of death, all the dramatic moments (fights, rapes, rejections, accidents, separations, humiliations, and so forth), have a geographical location in the universe relative to the planets and other systems. These positions are associated by the brain with the individual's feelings and are memorized by the body. When the brain detects its position in space, it can bring from the depths the memory of the excessive distress associated with that position. Furthermore, for information carved in a solid manner, for example on a slab of marble, time's effects are minimal. Rain, sun, cold, and the passing years do not affect the information.

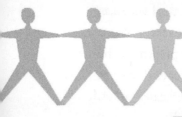

TWELVE

TRANSGENERATIONAL PROGRAMMING

Every lie places us "outside reality." To be outside reality is the same as being dead.

ELISABETH HOROWITZ,
Se libérer du destin familial
(FREEDOM FROM YOUR FAMILY DESTINY)

Every part of a tree exists in ceaseless interdependence with its other parts. A tree does not live to make branches and leaves; to the contrary, it creates branches and leaves so that it may live.

In identical fashion, animal and human lines project themselves into the future. They make children in order to live, but they do not live for the purpose of making children. The parents, the ancestors (dead or alive), are always present, living in memory in the family tree, just as in real trees, the branches and trunk are always there, stems that have lengthened and grown larger over the years, features of the union between the past and the future.

Consequently, resolving what remains unresolved from the past is a completely natural action for the biological brain, as the sap that circulates inside carries a significant amount of information. Past, present, and future combine as one at every instant. The past is there, grown hardened and ligneous; the present is the bark bordering the future; and past and present already have, in their sketchbooks, the outlines and blueprints for the branches and leaves of the coming spring.

When the body manufactures a tumor or some other kind of disorder, it is not responding to the neutral reality of a single moment, nor is the automatic pilot doing so when it guides the individual to make this or that professional or emotional choice. However, both are clearly reacting to memories (ancient realities, or what were interpreted to be realities in an earlier time) that have been left by the individual's ancestors. Because of civil wars, wars between nations, economic and religious crises, and incomprehensible shocks—and the neuroses they create—there are countless varieties of unresolved conflicts centered on guilt, shame, frustration, and other secret family skeletons. Anything that applies pressure to the individual—political or religious doctrines, wars with their parades of death, violence or humiliation of all kinds, arbitrary abuse and injustice, bastard children who are kept hidden—conditions the person, restricts possibilities, and prevents him or her from reacting freely.

The person's suffering settles in for a long stay if the values or taboos of the person's surroundings encourage this. The death of a loved one often crushes plans for the future, extinguishes innocence and dreams, and creates shortcomings and desires that leap over a generation to the next one (children who take the father's place, who take care of their younger siblings), creating mental confusion. Guilt over the inability to do anything to save someone close to a person can haunt the following generations and thus program conflicts for them (muscular pathologies, pulmonary and blood disorders, cerebral and thyroid disorders, and so forth).

Robert had a leg amputated at Verdun and had a passionate affair with the nurse who cared for him, but this liaison had no future because he was already married. When his granddaughter was eighteen, despite her parents' objections, she entered nursing school, where she became a specialist in cardiology. Robert's granddaughter "sacrificed" herself to bring into the family tree the nurse who had created such a huge void in the life of her grandfather.

A mother died while giving birth to her daughter, Felice. The shock to the family was quite difficult to bear, and the memory of the event and everything it brought about was transmitted into the family unconscious. This prepared the terrain for Beatrice, a descendant two generations later, to be childless and living alone at the age of forty-six. Because the event had created the perception that giving birth was dangerous, celibacy, sterility, or abortion were all solutions that the autonomic unconscious brain determined were crucial to survival.

Alphonse died during World War I from poison gas during the battle of Verdun. One of his grandchildren and two of his great-grandchildren suffered from asthma. The body's autonomic solution to avoid death was to not breathe, preventing the gas from entering the lungs.

The earthworms of the famous Dr. Pavlov, which were stuck with a needle in the presence of light, gave birth to descendants who had clearly integrated the behavioral solution of their parents to this problem. They squirmed and twisted away when exposed to light (light = pain).

Henri was the eldest child. He was deported to Germany, where he died. His brother, Andrew, had to assume the heavy burden of being the family's lone male survivor, along with the guilty feeling, "Why him and not me?" He had five children. The eldest died the day following his birth. His third child, Roger, conceived four children, the first of whom died in a miscarriage; his fourth child, a daughter, died when she was nineteen. Roger's second and third children both resorted to abortions to get rid of their first pregnancies. Over three generations, the eldest born (the fourth child corresponds to the oldest child) died. Initially, in the family imprint, the disappearance of the oldest child had caused a problem. The solution: Have no more oldest children.

Anita (the second child) found herself widowed with three children to raise. She obtained a job as a canteen worker at a police barracks and also found work harvesting grapes and picking olives. Her granddaughter (also a second-born child), who was named Juanita, manufactured a breast cancer. This cancer (whose meaning is to symbolically prepare a woman to provide better nourishment to a significant other by providing more nutritious milk) was the biological solution to the excessive distress experienced by her grandmother when confronted with the necessity of feeding three children by herself. A study of the memorized cellular cycles of Juanita shows that the formation of her cancer also arose in tune with an event of her childhood, when she thought German police had imprisoned her mother.

It Is Elementary

The logic used by nature to provide a solution to the problems it encounters is a very simple, even primary logic. If greed was the culprit in the creation of an excessive stress, one or more descendants may live in utter poverty or sacrifice themselves endlessly without receiving any compensation. If the loss of a child or children who died too soon has created great distress, the descendants will not have any children, or perhaps only a few. Women might create uterine fibroids in symbolic compensation, or have very intense premenstrual symptoms or hemorrhaging.

We should note here that the appearance of either a physical or a mental illness, or a particular life destiny, does not erase the programming that called it into being. So if Janine became paralyzed when she was twenty-two, it does not mean that no one descended from her will ever create a paralysis. Only conscious realization (or a long period spanning generations and thus much sacrifice) of the original excessive stress will permit Janine and her descendants to erase the program.

This means we must understand the ancestor's excessive distress, integrate it, and then resolve it by means other than through the use of our organs or our destiny (through metaphorical actions, for example). Only this enables the individual to heal and also to free other descendants, even if these latter descendants have not undertaken a similarly proactive approach.

Kirk was an adventurer who owned nothing but who frequented the company of real estate agents and notaries. As a youth, he worked in a stable yard and owned a horse. He learned, much later, that his great-grandfather had once traded horses, unaware that they had been stolen. His grandfather was falsely accused of the crime and spent time in prison. Later in life, the grandfather entrusted his fortune to a dishonest notary who ruined him. The equation "possession leads to dispossession, shame, and prison" set the stage for three of his descendants, one of whom was Kirk, to feel uncomfortable owning things. As a result, they shunned ownership of possessions, getting by with as few material goods during their lives as possible.

Unwittingly, we choose our spouse to reveal something to us about our family tree. Gabriel was engaged to a woman who had been raped in her own home when she was eighteen. (Her mother had also been debased and assaulted.) Gabriel's fiancée spent much of her time washing the carpets, the quilts, and the curtains, as if seeking to wash out the stain. It so happens that Gabriel's grandmother had also been raped when she was young. Gabriel's fiancée revealed to him, through her compulsive ritualistic behavior, something he did not yet know about his own ancestors and something he could see in himself, a biological conflict around the theme of debasement or being soiled, which he had inherited.

Secrets

Quite often, events that are difficult to confess have been hidden and remain concealed in the family past.

For instance, a woman's statement, "I cannot *say* whether or not this child is my husband's," programs illnesses affecting the oropharynx and the jaw. To talk, it is first necessary to "open up," and it is the bones of the jaw that open the mouth so that the vocal cords can emit intelligible sounds.

That Luigi was cheated of his family inheritance through his brother's manipulations programs depressions, renal and pancreatic disorders, and decalcification of the vertebrae and ribs of some of Luigi's descendants.

Regrettable events, crimes, thefts, despoilment, incest, and rape are often hidden by the majority of the members of a family in a consensus whose purpose is to spare sensitive souls shame and embarrassment. From one generation to the next, the event is locked in the closet, or its narrative is altered. But the original painful and conflicted feeling continues on its course, silently leaping from generation to generation, where it is transmuted into illnesses or behaviors (to have no abilities at math or history, to be confused, stammer, be dyslexic, be suicidal, fail financially, and so on). Because there are entire sections of logic lacking in the ideas one has of one's family, the mystery compels the descendants to feel abnormal, inferior, or cursed.

When a painful reality has been disguised and lies have coated over the facts, when social conventions, shame, or pride have brought about exclusions (those who are absent are always wrong), we tend to idealize the miscreants. An idealized vision of a deceased spouse may be established, for instance, or parents who were liars and usurpers are transformed into heroes.

One's descendants seek, without being aware of it, to resemble ancestors who, in fact, behaved horribly, or condemn others ("Your father abandoned us") who, in fact, were victims. If I lie in a recurrent and compulsive manner, it means a huge family secret exists that is related to what I lie *about*. For the heir, the secret is like a ball and chain, which makes it extremely difficult to get at the truth. Thus, over the span of several generations, we see the repeated occurrence of identical conflicts and identical illnesses.

Repetition

But this repetition is not merely a punitive mechanism that, once started, is hard to keep under control. The purpose of transgenerational transmission is clearly to forewarn. Through individual behavior or a physical anomaly, the descendants are alerted to the problem, and this helps them adapt so that the line of which they are a part can triumph in a battle lost at an earlier time. It is a principle of precaution based on the assumption that what happened once could recur thirty, eighty, or even one hundred and twenty years later. Nature functions analogically. This is why situations seem to repeat, generation upon generation, cycle after cycle, in the same way that the planets of our solar system appear to us to move in cycles.

A woman is humiliated, and the tone of her humiliation is deeply etched into the family lineage. Her daughter or her granddaughter develops this tonality by placing herself in a position to be humiliated by or to humiliate others.

The child who has been victimized by a pedophile, as a kind of emergency exit from the obsessive feeling of being his aggressor's property, may himself develop a tendency to spend time with those who are younger than he is. And he may also touch children in an inappropriate way so as to no longer feel alone in his distress.

THIRTEEN

THE UNKNOWING PARENTAL PROJECTION

Being born within a family, is another way of
saying "one is possessed!"

ALEXANDRO JODOROWSKI,
Le Théâtre de la guérison
(THE THEATER OF HEALING)

The practice of biogenealogical exploration reveals that the mother's life story resembles that of the father's.

Everything starts with a meeting. A man and woman are attracted to each other because their brains have detected a certain complementary relationship between the life experiences of their respective ancestors, the former lives of these two individuals. This similarity or complementary nature is also manifest in their birth charts. This meeting of two symbolic twins can be like a stroke of lightning, with kisses that give off sparks.

The romantic liaison is analogous to the bonding of molecules, which is only possible if the couple's geometric structures are compatible; if the energy that gives them life makes them sufficiently strongly attracted to each other; and if they approach from the appropriate angle when this meeting occurs.

During the initial meeting, the two brains quickly grasp whether this liaison will be propitious for births and the settling of one or more old scores, and what opportunities each individual gives the other to evolve, among other factors. The choice of a spouse for procreative purposes is also subordinate to a mutual inventory of genes that is established unbeknownst to either of the two people.

The fact is that when two individuals are next to each other, their brains are comparing their respective chromosomes. A test was conducted in which young girls were asked to select their preferred odor from among T-shirts that had been worn by men. Each female was drawn to the odor of the man who was genetically the most different from her. When choosing between a complete similarity and a total dissimilarity of genes, the brain prefers difference over similarity, in obedience to the archaic principle of complementary experiences to increase the chances of survival. But it also seems that if there is a choice between an individual offering a small amount of genetic similarity and one who is completely different in this regard, the brain opts for the partner that offers a small degree of similarity.

The meeting of an individual's parents had a place and a date. The child's blueprint was therefore already "out in the ether" even if the parents were not aware of it. This "ether" carries the shortcomings of each family tree. Each is asking the other to compensate for his or her lacks. This is analogous to the character in Molière's *Le Malade Imaginaire* who wanted his daughter to marry the son of a physician, so he could have a doctor in the house who would treat his illnesses.

Even if the parents consciously desire to avoid having children, the sap of the family tree is running, and fertilization can take place if it is "written" in their respective trees. Every child is strongly desired by the two trees that combine to make his or her specific genealogy. This can be comforting to know. The trees of our gardens "know" to the exact degree how many leaves they will sprout and how many fruits they will carry the following spring.

The Ambience of Fertilization

At the moment of conception, the problems of both parents due to the memories of excessive stresses in the family trees, their unease, their anxieties, their struggles, their happiness, their shame, their guilt, their regret, their insecurity, their neuroses, the things they hide from others, the things they hide from themselves—all leave their mark on the child.

Anastasia was pregnant by her husband, with whom she was no longer getting along, when she met and fell in love with Boris. But when Boris learned that Anastasia was pregnant by her husband, he broke off the relationship. Anastasia was deeply distressed by this. Twenty-two years later, her daughter was suffering from depression, isolating herself in her room with just the television for company. She had no plans for the future, no friends, no husband, and no children. The essential factor that programmed this depression and sterility was the message: The child comes accompanied by separation and sorrow.

A child might be desired to serve as the glue between the members of a couple, but does that ensure that the child will be loved? One of the parents might want a child as a means of holding onto a partner who is seeking to leave. At conception, the child born from this kind of union receives the information that movement is dangerous and, as a result, may be born paralyzed or develop paralysis during the course of his or her life; or the child may experience mental paralysis on a regular basis when confronted with conflicting options.

Jean-Jacques was in love with a woman named Jeanine, who

died after being struck by a car. Later he married another woman, with whom he had a son. This son became enthusiastic about driving and was a fan of auto racing (mastering the car and the trajectory of its movement is an *a posteriori* solution to this kind of conflict).

Hervé was born in 1942. His father was sent to Austria to fulfill his STO* so that his son could be eligible for a free milk ration. Hervé's father returned at the end of the war, leaving behind a woman with whom he had had an amorous liaison.

Hervé's life had depended on the milk and thus on the loss of his father's freedom; then it depended on the return of his father, which necessitated the loss of his father's relationship with his lover. Hervé was faithful, without knowing it, to the type of events that had allowed him to grow up, and as a result was incapable of maintaining a durable relationship as part of a couple. He thus found himself alone for the most part because of the equation that had been unknowingly established for him. That equation was as follows: Conjugal love and love for a child bring about the loss of freedom; when freedom is restored, it brings about the loss of love and joy.

When Hervé was fifty, he had an automobile accident as he was leaving his father's property. He fractured his wrist (symbolic of imprisonment, handcuffs, and forced labor) and dislocated his hip (symbolic of obstructed sexuality), which prompted the revelation of his father's unspoken conflicts.

During Annie's pregnancy, her mother learned of the death of her brother in a tropical jungle. The joy Annie was feeling as an expectant mother had no outlet, as she was forced into the role of consoling her mother and thus had to contain her feelings. All her life, Annie felt deprived of joy, manufacturing a case of

---

*STO, or Service du Travail Obligatoire, was a work program established by the Nazis.

hyperglycemia whose conflict was repugnance (due to the strong emotion felt by her mother when imagining her brother's decomposed body).

Again, a poem will help to illustrate the text.

Fox and Vixen

A fox and a vixen met
During a particularly harsh winter.
Famished, they found refuge and sustenance
In a cellar where cheeses were aged.
This took place in the Savoy region.
This was where they coupled. A fox kit was born
Who became an expert in the art of attracting crows to
*   him*
Who carried a piece of cheese in their beaks . . .

The old unresolved conflicts of our ancestors and the emotions experienced by our parents during the perigestational period are imprinted onto the child. Marc Fréchet has devoted much of his attention to this idea of parental impression. (This impression is now more commonly known as *meaning unconsciously projected by the parents*, but I prefer the term *unknowing parental projection,* as I feel it is more accurate.)

A projection is a form of transfer. To borrow an analogy from the film world, whatever is inscribed on film is what is projected on the screen. The film has been given an impression by an earlier experience: the scene played by the actors. Our reality could be a kind of hologram (a three-dimensional reproduction based on information that has been recorded in our cellular memory).

The projection onto the child is unknowing; neither of the parents, in the normal course of things, has any real awareness of the scenario being imprinted on the film that is the future child.

The annunciations made to Mary and Elizabeth could be prime

examples of unknowing parental projection. Couldn't the conception of Jesus and John the Baptist by way of the Word and an angel highlight this invisible downloading of a blueprint, one containing various scenarios and already sketched-out life plans that we are now discovering?

To those of my readers who believe reincarnating souls come from deceased individuals who were not family members, who were strangers, let me point out that from around the year 1000 to the present day (a figure that would equal approximately thirty-four generations before us), each of us should have more than four billion ancestors. It so happens that in the year 1000 there were not even close to that many people on the planet, and this is not even taking into account remarriages and extramarital relationships. We are all cousins, more or less in tune with one another and therefore all more or less capable of taking on missions coming from every point of the immense family of humanity.

The child's life includes, as prescribed by its particular scenario, incidents of happiness, or, conversely, illnesses, depression, jobs for which he or she is ill-suited, gifts and talents, relationships with people with whom he or she cannot get along, and so on. If a person cannot find happiness as a member of a couple, it may be due, for example, to the person's parents having married out of spite (unrequited love or a failure to find a better spouse), or to one of the parents having spent his or her life regretting the loss of an earlier love. The biological solution to avoid this kind of suffering is to refrain from loving, or to give one's love to an imaginary and therefore nonexistent person (the myth of the ideal woman or perfect man).

Our suffering is the result of overcompensation by our safety mechanisms and an overdose of analogy.

The Intrauterine Period

Dr. Alfred Tomatis tells us in his book on uterine life, *La Nuit Uterine* (The Uterine Night), that the eggs of singing birds, if hatched by nonsinging birds, produce birds that do not sing. This speaks volumes about the importance of the information that is transmitted between the parents and the child during the "hatching" period, in other words, during pregnancy.

The brain of the fetus establishes equations based on everything it perceives. If the embryo feels it is a problem for its mother, it either grows larger as if to confirm its existence, or shrinks as if to disappear. Researchers have provided convincing evidence that the fetus is already thinking by six months after conception, if not sooner. The fetus also feels any earlier excessive stress that has been experienced by the uterus (abortions, miscarriages).

Twin pregnancies are fairly frequent, but both twins are not always brought to term. Sometimes one of the two embryos, after growing to the size of one or two millimeters, disappears. In such a case, the other keenly feels that death and separation and, later in life, feels a sense of unconscious guilt whose origin cannot easily be traced back to its source. The person feels an obligation to live two lives at the same time.

What the parents and those in their immediate surroundings say, even anecdotally, can take on some importance for the child *in utero*. The child adopts, without the ability to analyze them, the parents' emotions, their stresses both small and large (the words of friends, neighbors, noises, and so on), and, later in life, may display a disorder or a problem connected to these stresses.

Strident sounds heard at the time the child's ears are in the budding stage programs hypersensitivity to noises later in life. The whine of a circular saw can awaken the archaic fear of wild animals, explains Dr. Hamer, and even bring about a clubfoot (this conflict's source is the wish to make oneself incapable of exiting the mother's belly).

Here is another example: During Frank's gestation, his mother was fighting with her husband because he refused to quit smoking. She would oppose her husband, then give up seeking to get her way, and then oppose him again, and on and on it went in this manner. As a result, the child displayed abnormalities in the lumbar vertebre because he had made his mother's emotional state (devaluation in opposition) his own.

Birth Is a Life-Shaping Experience

The biological conflicts of the family tree that are related to lines of descent—sexuality, incest, and rape—could set the stage for labor that can be abnormally long, painful, and problematic. These memories create muscular tensions or motor breakdowns that prevent the baby from emerging because there may be an unconscious desire to take revenge on the ancestor whom the baby will replace. The pelvic channel engraves messages on the baby as it is passing through, in much the same way that a laser engraves music or data on CD-ROMs.

Then there is the trauma of the birth itself. This can include the transformation of the birth experience into an over-medicalized procedure: administering drugs to accelerate or delay labor and to anesthetize, placing the mother in a horizontal position, using forceps to pull the baby out, and so on—all colored by the mother's fear of the medical personnel. It also includes the welcome given the newborn: harsh operating room lights, chilly temperatures, noise, cutting the umbilical cord too soon, taking the baby away from the mother for several moments, or more often hours or even days. These are all contributing factors that can add more suffering to the trials the infant has already experienced in its journey to its destiny in the open air.

The moment of birth is sacred, because it is unique. Being born can be the most traumatic experience an individual may ever have to go through to live. After around nine months within the closed vessel of the mother's uterus, in a placenta that confers safety and security, what the child experiences during this passage into the world sets the tone and provides the ambience for the rest of its life.

Konrad Lorenz was one of the modern discoverers of the phenomenon of imprinting. His experiments with geese are now famous. As most will recall, he found that if what baby geese first saw after breaking out of their eggs was a human being, they would consider that human their mother and not let him or her move more than a step away from them without following.

The moment when the progeny sees the day is a time and space in which everything that is experienced at that moment is primordially imprinted and sets the tone for that individual's life. Furthermore, apprenticeship is particularly facilitated at this time of life, because the nervous system is still under construction, and neurons are being produced in great quantity. The baby has its "window wide open," fitting comfortably into what will henceforth be its surroundings. Newborn babies greedily extend their senses toward the life surrounding them, memorizing all they can perceive. The mother's uterine walls have been replaced by the air, air that seems to have no boundaries.

An intrepid explorer landed on an island and was captured and tortured by its native inhabitants. He finally managed to escape, putting an end to what had been a period of great tension. This unfortunate experience had become imprinted and, subsequently, his autonomic brain maintained a "state of war," a state of vigilance, even if the danger was nonexistent, every time he set his feet on the ground. He would even create conflict-filled situations of great tension as justification for his vigilant state and to exorcise his earlier sufferings. This was because his brain had established the equation that in order to survive, tension was necessary, and after tension dissipated, freedom would appear.

The way in which one is born shapes the personality. Unfortunately, birth can be a long, drawn-out process of anguish, pain, anoxia, and suffering that the baby is incapable of analyzing, dispelling, or understanding. A baby who has been indirectly anesthetized because of the drugs given to dull its mother's labor pains can feel powerless to leave the womb by its own steam and asks for help by falling back into sleep and torpor. This individual will become an adult who finds it impossible to be prepared and advance on his or her own; the person will be dependent on others. The memory of the anesthesia becomes an insidious force inside, sapping the person's strength.

The stored-up energy of natal suffering accumulates in the parts of the brain that are capable of storing it at that age. Like all energy, it seeks to express itself, to come to life, often without the individual's awareness. This kind of experience sets the stage for excessive caution, difficult reactions, beliefs that are wrong because they are obsolete, and/or relational, professional, or sexual difficulties.

American statistics have shown that close to 100 percent of criminals, fanatics, and terrorists had a very traumatic birth, which was followed by a childhood characterized by a lack of love. Obviously, no mother is responsible for her way of giving birth. Mothers do the best they can with the genealogical burdens they have inherited. Deprogramming and a greater awareness of the intricacies of one's family tree can make difficult labors the exception and not the rule. Furthermore, as Frederic Leboyer* proposes, encouraging labor and birth without violence is a solution to the problems of a hard life.

---

*Frederic Leboyer is an advocate of natural childbirth and the gentle treatment of babies during and after birth; he wrote the bestseller *Birth Without Violence*.

Postnatal Life

A child has appeared. Not only does it shake its parents' world, but by offering a new springtime to its lineage, it causes the entire, still-growing family tree to tremble, soothed by this new being who will assume several of the missions that are part of the tree's dynamic. The child makes the third point of a triangle that it inaugurates with its parents. Depending on whether the child feels it is a source of joy to its parents, it reacts with different resources.

At every stage of development, with every conflict, the child utilizes the resources acquired earlier. The child learns to play with the mental world of its parents and to use their poles of interest to act upon them. In return, as "feedback," the parents react in accordance with their interpretation, their genealogical lexicon of meaning, and their beliefs. Things that we consider terrible can result from this interlinking (autism, violent behavior, crying, blackmail, "What a plague this kid is!"), as well as things we consider terrific (resiliency, laughter, and griefs that are over as soon as they appear). (For more on this, the works of Françoise Dalto are very informative, as well as Boris Cyrulnik's book, *Les vilains petits canards* [Ugly Ducklings].)

At the various stages of childhood development (oral, anal, Ocdipal), the dramas that can arise in a child's life, such as separation from the mother or the arrival too soon of a little brother or a little sister, produce specific behaviors and symptoms (bulimia during the oral stage; constipation during the anal stage) that can last an entire lifetime. During the first great distress experienced in its life, the child will perceive a strategy enabling it to obtain what it needs. It will subsequently, for the rest of its life, make use of this same strategy (for example, to attract attention and to be of service so as not to be ignored) in every occasion. This is an effective strategy nine times out of ten.

FOURTEEN

WHERE, WHEN, AND HOW?

The individual who had to fight to be born will arrange things later in life so that everything becomes a fight.

ARTHUR JANOV, *Imprints*

Where? The Itinerary of the Programming

In a tree—a pine tree, for example—what vibrates in unison with the trunk of the tree is the new bark of the year. What vibrates in unison with last year's leaves are the leaves of the new year. And what vibrates with an ancestor fruit and its concerns as a fruit is definitely the new fruit of the year.

Inside the line of the Dupont family, it seems that only the descendants who vibrate in unison with a particular ancestor will be able to resolve the problem or problems left behind by that ancestor. This is how, in a totally logical fashion, the memories of prior difficult life experiences are transmitted. This is why the children of one couple are different from one another. Although they share the same blood and the same ancestors, they have different destinies.

Each child holds a specific place in the brother/sister group and family pecking order (the eldest, the second-born, the youngest) and can inherit programs from an ancestor who occupied the same spot in the generational hierarchy.

Furthermore, each child arrives at a distinct moment in the lives of its parents. From one child to the next, the parents often evolve, at least in one domain, be it material, sexual, emotional, intellectual, or spiritual. At the time of each conception, the desires and expectations of the parents may be different from what they were when previous children were conceived. The world the parents live in influences them; various regional, national, and global events have an impact on their lives.

One or more people close to the parents may die around the time of conception. The name or names given to the child, if they are taken from the family tree, represent this ancestor to society again. This explains why brothers and sisters do not share the same destiny, why some succeed with seemingly no effort and others toil thanklessly or fail. The unknowing parental projections are different, as are the ancestors whose influence is felt. Children conceived during difficult times in the parents' lives have more problems than those conceived during times of joy and prosperity.

When? The Moment Something Manifest Appears

Problems and illnesses, like happier events, arrive at precise times in the individual's life; they are predetermined. Imagine for a moment if the memories of our own difficulties, those of our parents, and those of our family tree were all expressed at the same time. The result would be pure chaos. To manufacture fifty illness solutions at one time would be fatal. Chronological order—each problem at its appointed time—is the winning solution for survival. This is why the brain reads these memories one after the other in a timely order, so it can resolve each of the problems in turn. If it is unable to resolve them in a conscious fashion, they will be displayed again cyclically, much as a bulge in a bike tire rubs the forks every time the wheel makes a complete revolution.

When an excessive distress, with its accompanying "feeling" has been memorized, it makes a cyclical appearance in the life of the descendant. It may appear once or twice without triggering the illness, but perhaps the third time will be the charm if the individual has not yet grasped the message and transmuted the energy.

It can transpire as if the emotion, at each turn of the wheel, stores away a little more of the kinetic energy thus generated before finally triggering a somatization. If we have not evolved in a timely manner by expressing our conflicts and letting go of them, the wheel of life claims a heavy price for our indigence. Marc Fréchet has given these cycles the name of "memorised cellular cycles."

The case history of Claude-Henri: "At birth I was separated from my mother and placed in an incubator. When I was eleven years old, my parents put me in a boarding school (it still hurts me to remember them walking away from the large staircase of the secondary school); at twenty-two I had to leave for the war in Indochina; at thirty-three years of age I saw my father fall off a ladder, and when I was fifty-five, my wife ran away with another man and my left leg became paralyzed" (the brain's solution to avoid going to boarding school or to war).

Witnessing the departure of his wife was highly traumatic for Claude-Henri, of course, as was leaving for the war, but it was much less distressing than being sent to boarding school when he was eleven, and even much less upsetting than his separation from his mother shortly after his birth. Of course, the episodes of excessive stress suffered at eleven and at birth would be among the factors considered by the therapist for healing the paralysis. But the one element that clearly emerges from this case is how Claude-Henri's destiny had an eleven-year rhythm.

The Corridors of Time

What makes an individual's pathological behavior, or that of one of the individual's organs (or even a lifestyle), inexplicable and abnormal to the eyes of an observer are the temporal boundaries of the context in which the observer is enclosed (quite naturally, of course).

For example, a young girl has a tic that causes her to project her head forcefully to one side. This behavior would be considered "pathological" because it would be inconsistent with the time and space parameters in the girl's life. It could be a solution to an experience she hadn't undergone personally. The event that is the source of this behavior can exist only in memory. The observer who, confronted with an individual stricken with a pathology, can borrow the person's corridor of time and discover, in the depths of the genealogical tree, the event that has brought it into being can help the patient heal.

The young girl with the tic was only realizing (in a loop) movement that had been prevented at an earlier time (during her life or the life of the ancestor) in the course of an oral rape, a movement that could have prevented the penetration.

Simply put, several years had elapsed between the initial event and its attempted resolution. Several elliptical orbits around the sun had occurred between the time of the event that had no solution and the time of the behavioral solution, between the cause and effect, between the ancestor experiencing excessive stress and her descendant. Because she inherited the information, she could bring about—*a posteriori* and compulsively, of course—the saving movement. It is the "temporal" shift and the chronicity of the behavior, of the illness, that makes it pathological.

A little girl was regularly forced to masturbate by her grandfather, and this disgusted her greatly. Once she had grown into adulthood, she gave birth to a boy whose penis was not completely developed.

The Transformation of an Event into Conflict

Among the millions of events that arise in the life of an individual, only certain events trigger conflicts. How it is that one person creates problems out of events that would not pose such issues for others is explained by these invisible programmings.

The emotional reactions are programmed, offering individuals a predetermination of their quality of life. The individual manufactures problems from everyday materials, but only if the prototypes of these problems are carried within.

In 1920, Gaspard, a cabinetmaker whose father was a stonecutter, planned to wed a young girl of nobility against the wishes of her parents. She was disinherited by her parents, both of whom died of grief several weeks before the wedding. After the wedding, Gaspard's wife cheated on him several times before abandoning him once and for all. The overriding emotion with which he experienced these events was one of betrayal. He would go to his deathbed still clinging to this state of mind.

The messages he left his descendants were: In life, one is betrayed by those one loves; and, love causes death. Two of his grandchildren made the same choices. They married women who, because the women had programming complementing that of their husbands, betrayed them so that they too could feel betrayal and experience a love that was impossible because it was fatal. Both grandchildren created depression, and one created sexual disorders to boot (prostate problems).

Nobody is truly the victim; nobody is truly guilty; each is using the other to reveal, during their lifetimes, feelings and emotions that are congealed within and have been congealed for a long time by the big chill that produced, among other things, "ancient" inflexible resources and limiting beliefs. Would you hate an actor whom you had engaged to play the role of a seducer who takes a spouse far away from the family hearth? Hasn't the script been written before the rehearsals take place? Isn't the actor merely inhabiting a role that he has been assigned to play?

So recurring problems exist that consume the family line's attention over the span of several generations. The first person who injects a distressful memory into the tree is obviously the individual who, caught on the wrong foot by a new kind of problem, is incapable of reacting. But every time a person is able to consciously resolve the problem of his or her tree, that person helps it to grow.

Clairvoyance and Foresight

We can always access this invisible programming, and one way to do this is to visit a "specialist of destiny," an individual who has a gift of clairvoyance and/or an understanding of astrology. A good astrologer knows how to decipher the symbolism of the planets at the time of an individual's birth, to understand the birth or to be able to deduce several delicate or favorable periods of that individual's future. Our lives are predetermined, therefore our future is already sketched out; and if we are incapable of erasing what has been drawn, the future will be achieved in accordance with the impetus of the past.

But the brain is also a computer with the ability to direct an individual toward realization and concretization of the predictions in which he or she has placed belief. Also, when clairvoyants and fortunetellers announce dark tidings of the future to their clients without explaining how they can manage these memories and these energies, they become dangerous. The fear of the thing to come brings about its arrival to help that fear disappear.

Someone who believes in the prediction acts to bring about its fulfilment. If the future that is foretold is good, fine; but if it is unfavorable, tragedy can result. In the myth of Oedipus, an oracle announced to King Laius that his son, Oedipus, would be the instrument of his death. Laius, gripped by fear, asked a servant to slay his son. But the servant was incapable of murdering the baby and entrusted it to some shepherds. When he had grown to adulthood, Oedipus left his homeland. While en route, he was verbally attacked by a man, Laius, whose chariot crushed one of Oedipus's feet. While Oedipus defended himself, Laius was dragged behind his horses and died. Would Oedipus have been the instrument of his father's death if his father had not believed the oracle's predictions? Probably not. Wasn't it the oracle's prediction and secrecy that set Oedipus on the same path as his parents?

The fear of a thing brings about its occurrence, whereas knowledge of the past makes it possible to react quite differently.

There Is Nothing New About This

Allusion is made in the Bible to this kind of transgenerational programming. In fact, it can be read in the Book of Exodus, chapter 20: "I am a jealous God, visiting the sins of the fathers upon the children, unto the third and fourth generation of those who hate me."

Also in the Bible, in Ezekiel, is the following verse: "The fathers eat sour grapes, and the children's teeth are set on edge," which can also be interpreted as, "The acidity of the ancestors' life will make that of their descendants acidic."

Abandoning the Conflict

Understanding transgenerational programming makes it possible to praise illness and destiny. While an illness or the repeated occurrence of disagreeable events in the life of an individual seems to have little justification, it is very easy to perceive its pertinence when we observe the life experiences of the individual's line (or end of the line), with all its dramas, tragedies, and unrealized hopes.

The system works quite well for the family line and much less so for the individual. But it is an old system that has accompanied every family line throughout all history up to our own time, and the challenge we now face is to learn how to transcend it and free ourselves from the restrictions that encumbered those who went before us. The child is enriched by the suffering of the elders and runs the risk of having his or her own life impoverished. But no piece of advice is too excessive for the line, which seeks its survival at any cost.

Bringing into our conscious awareness the experiences our ancestors lived through, and grasping what has programmed our fortunes and misfortunes, our joys and sorrows, is not the equivalent of condemning or accusing our ancestors. It is through understanding that we are able to heal and evolve. There are no guilty parties. Once we are informed of the real state of things, there are no grounds for bringing accusations against our ancestors. The most we can do is attack the transgenerational mechanism itself.

Our life has been drawn out and is already defined, but this is not a question of holding our ancestors responsible for everything that happens over the course of our lives. Once we have been taught about this transgenerational process, we are a little more alive, a little more active, and a little more aware. Our ability to act on our own destiny then begins to grow like a frail sprout carving its way toward the light.

The loyalty we always show toward our family tree and our ancestors (even if we think we detest them) therefore often proves problematic, simply because we are not at all aware of it. We have no idea this loyalty exists and what it makes us do. What is this loyalty based on? It is the reassuring attraction it offers of safety and security. A sense of isolation and the feeling of being completely alone are the greatest threats an individual can encounter. We need the group, the clan, for our protection (in union there is strength), to hunt, to protect what we have laid claim to, to have direction.

It so happens that the primordial membership of an individual is within his or her family tree. A tree is a source of protection that can also feed the person living in it. Before forming bonds with friends, classmates, fellow soldiers, and fellow workers, before we start promoting and developing the qualities that make us different, we are woven by our family tree. It just so happens that this family tree, which has known episodes of excessive stress, trials, and losses, gives off a distinct aura. It has an ambience that becomes the reference for all other references.

This ensures that at every crossroads we come to in our individual lives, when opportunities for taking new roads are presented to us, what we hear most loudly is that loyalty to our family tree. Evolution, therefore, raises the question: Who is commanding this ship? This job I have chosen, is it my true vocation, something that will make me happy? Or is it, to the contrary, a choice I have made due to unwitting loyalty to my family tree? ("My two grandmothers were servants, and I do housework"; "My two great-grandfathers were captains of industry, and I am studying company management courses.")

Let's say, for example, that there is a young woman, my uncle's maid, with whom I have conceived a child. Did I truly choose her of my own volition, or was the choice made for me by my family tree (because her family tree resembled mine), so as to reveal an ancillary extramarital relationship of a great-grandfather, one that resulted in the birth of a child, whose existence was kept a secret from the family?

Or, let's say I am planning to take a position as a teacher in the state educational system after the recent failure of my business, but I wonder whether the failure was due to my own incompetence, or was the result of an equation manufactured by my family tree ("My great-grandparents separated at the time they were running a business together"). The question is, to remain part of a couple, is it necessary to avoid becoming a salesman or merchant?

The initiatory quest that allows us to evolve proceeds through the clarification and illumination of these loyalties that feel so reassuring. Giving ourselves permission to think differently from our family of origin, and understanding that while we cannot change others, we can change ourselves, our reality, and our world, we can become who we truly are. These, and ceasing to be judgmental, are the means that allow us access to this extremely desirable state governed by free will. The gaze we train on our destiny or on our illness can, in fact, be our chief stumbling block. So it is already a fine thing to know how to accept what is, and it is an equally fine thing to be able to confidently visualize what we want.

> *It is not the intense emotions*
> *Of which we are aware*
> *But those we have forgotten,*
> *And those, occulted,*
> *Of our genealogical tree*
> *That make*
> *Our illnesses and destinies.*
> *If this was not in fact the case,*
> *Why then we would have already*
> *Cured*
> *Our illnesses and destinies.*

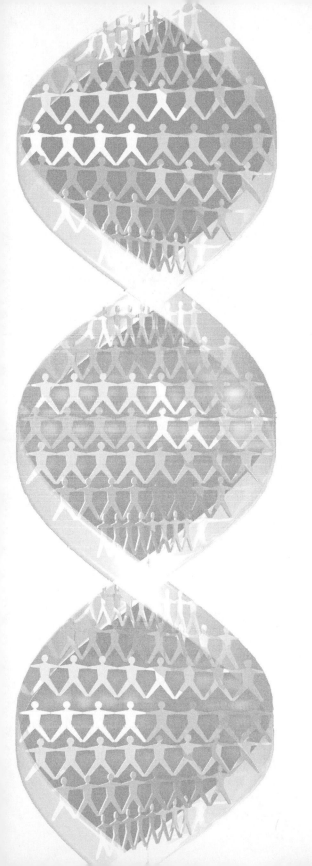

PART THREE

IMAGINE

FIFTEEN

A THERAPEUTIC PATH

Whether the objective is healing someone of a clinically abnormal behavior, of an undesirable effect of destiny, or of
an illness, or whether it is strictly a preventive measure, the manner of proceeding is always the same. Likewise, healing a group, a
people, or a nation of problematic behaviors is carried out by the
same kind of therapeutic investigation.

Process of Illness and the Self-Cure

Memorized distressful information + catalyzing event

Physical or behavioral disorder, lifestyle

Realization, contrary information

Cure

Figure 15.1

When life allows us to concretely resolve a conflict—and this happens quite often—we are not always aware of what was in play

(a problem from childhood, or one even older inherited from the family tree), and the conflict can make an appearance again later. On the other hand, a resolution that is made with full awareness of the programming involved, with evolution and a return to reality, is the equivalent of weeding a garden in which the unwanted plants are pulled up by the roots. These plants will not grow back.

As long as a piece of information has not been erased, it can present itself anew. Excessive distress may be as old as two hundred years, but it still can come back to life in a moment, and it is always potentially ready to reappear. The shock experienced by the individual becomes the catalyst (activator) of the adaptive reaction (the cold illness), and the contrary event, or the pressure of the therapist, becomes the catalyst (facilitator) of the reparative reaction. Over the space of the last several years, this has brought about the emergence of a therapeutic modality whose axis is the search for and erasure of the information responsible for the origin of the illness.

In fact, two modalities coexist today. One is the "medicine of effects," which seeks to treat the symptoms or effects of illness; the other is a "medicine of causes," which is what we have been discussing all along. While these two modalities revolve around the same reality, they are not currently in the same orbit. Humanity would gain greatly if they could be combined.

Treating the Cause

While treatments of symptoms have their applications when the resolution of a conflict or getting beyond it proves difficult, impossible, or dangerous, the therapeutic objective consists now of seeking, and helping the patient find, the right information (a feeling for his specific case. Starting from a precise medical diagnosis established by standard check-up procedures (such as blood tests, urine analyses, the X-rays of organs and so forth), or established by other kinds of examinations (such as brain scans, iridology readings, energy readings, blood protein tests, etc.) and through a knowledge of the process of illness and the role played by each kind of tissue and the symbolism of each organ and its function, the therapist-decoder can find the nature of the intense feeling that caused the illness.

Light and Darkness

The door is narrow. There is a very specific piece of information that will tip the scales toward healing. What prevents healing is lack of information about the conflict that is hanging on, waiting to be resolved. What needs to be done is to find the feeling of distress, along with its spatial and temporal context. And this is sometimes a difficult task, for people find it easy to forget, as a form of self-protection.

In the writings of the disciple Luke, Jesus explains the effect of occultation, of "unconscious repression" on health: "Your eye is the lamp of your body. When your eye is sound your entire body is full of light, but when your eye is not sound, your body is full of darkness" (Luke 11:33–36). Every individual in conflict has a small zone of this window that is opaque, preventing the light of awareness from passing through. There is an aberrational moment, a moment of forgetfulness and confusion concerning the individual's perception of his or her history and present. The individual does not see certain things that others are sometimes capable of seeing. The individual cannot see the old origin of the problem; he or she is too far from the reality and is living in illusion.

The Importance of the Gaze of the Other

To be cured of a physical manifestation of a conflict, whether it is a stomach ache, a breast cancer, sterility, a tendency to be disorganized, falling in love with people who are already spoken for, resorting to an abortion, manufacturing eczema, creating sprains or too much stomach gas, having car accidents, painful periods, or hot flashes, or dislocating a rib, it is necessary to identify the problem for which this manifestation—you guessed it—is the solution.

To do this we require the gaze of another. If we wish to find for ourselves the information frozen in our own dark "Great North," we go looking where there is already some light. To do that, we borrow the paths already traced in our brains. The journey does not lead us straight to the goal, as it is not the intense emotions we are aware of that trigger illnesses or other manifestations, but those which have been forgotten.

It is difficult to be one's own therapist. As author Jean-Yves Leloup puts it so well, "To go toward oneself one needs the gaze of the other." I cannot be aware of the tree concealed behind me except for the intermediary provided by the gaze of the other. The other is a mirror that brings the forest of the ancestors into view, the forest that hides itself behind the tree that I am and which guides my steps. This other may be a friend, a husband, the milkman, a bartender, in fact any person that lends attention. This person perceives some kind of conflict in me, through the sound of my voice, the words I use, my intonation, my gestures, my requests, and so on, and gives it back to me in a form I can reintegrate. The other is like a transformer that lowers the tension of the electricity, enabling it to be received and used.

In the same way, the biological-decoder therapist is a mirror who leads the patient to his or her hidden memory, to the zone of repressed content that corresponds to the problem. The therapist oversees the patient's progress to ensure he or she finds a way out of the illusion and takes a stand at a "yes" or a "no," no longer vacillating between them. It is a question of exiting the illusion, exiting the idea the person has painted of the situation, and returning to the neutral reality.

The ability of therapist-decoders to be sensitive listeners, their powers of observation, enables them to exploit every clue that spills from our unconscious when we consult with them. The events of our lives, illnesses, repeating dates, corresponding figures, street names, family names, first names, professions, posture, the gestures accompanying our words, miniature caresses and tiny scratching movements, gaps, recurring or incongruent words, the names, professions, and illnesses of our friends, the breaking of everyday objects, the illnesses of domestic animals, inconsistencies in the perception of the chronology of events, things forgotten and overlooked, dreams, nightmares, hesitations, silences, abnormalities in the curve of our voice's frequencies—all indicate our programming and triggering instants.

The Investment of the Consultant

Healing ourselves of a manifestation once and for all, and eradicating it within, involves a transformation of the inner landscape, a letting go. Keeping hold of something requires a great deal of tension and effort and causes a loss of energy that prevents attainment of the goal. Letting go is simply dropping the difficulty. The cure sometimes depends on a confession, a granting of forgiveness, a mourning period brought to a close, an acceptance, a firm decision, and a eureka-like moment of discovery concerning the meaning of the experience that has been lived. How many women who found it impossible to get pregnant have become mothers simply by letting go of their tense and overwrought desire?

What befalls a person as a result may be the materialization of the plan that the brain has crafted; it is a self-fulfilling prophecy. As a consequence, it is possible to heal if the person is convinced it is possible (think of the immense power of the placebo effect). The patient who understands the divine plan of the illness knows that he or she can heal, and this soothing certainty, by saving energy, leads to a cure. In order to avoid recreating the illness in the future, an internal conversion could be necessary, and this conversion is easier to undertake if its intimate functioning has been uncovered, and if one learns how to expand the context in which one has allowed oneself to become imprisoned.

Procedures of Therapeutic Approach

1. *Gain awareness of the existence of the problematic manifestation.* This may appear to be obvious, but numerous cold abnormalities of the body are invisible and painless. When the manifestation that is the problem involves a behavior (a fear, a loyalty, for example), it is often even harder to perceive.
2. *Set up an appointment with a therapist.* The brain, at this precise moment, records the goal of evolving and healing. The cure begins at this very moment.
3. *The therapist explains illness, destiny, and what is the biological meaning of the trouble.*
4. *Search for the intense emotion responsible for the manifestation.* Pushing the individual seeking consultation to bring the emotion into awareness is the first phase of therapy. This is in no way an intellectual quest. The therapist launches a search, and when the feeling is newfound—flooded by the light of consciousness and put in relation to the manifestation by new brain cabling—frees the blocked energy to temporarily erase the conflict. In a second phase, the therapist decoder helps the patient to bring solutions to his biological conflicts in order to definitively stop the symptoms. Then, the therapist researches the earlier programming conflict (from the individual's childhood, from the period around birth, and, if the patient knows his ancestors, in his genealogical tree).
5. *The cure of an illness can be immediate (under 2 or 3 days) or gradual, or it can go through a hot phase.* When the cure of a cold

illness goes through a painful hot phase, which can be characterized by edemas, inflammations, and infections, it is in the best interests of the patient that he or she understand what is happening. If the patient has completely integrated the knowledge that the hot phase is clearly a repair, there is no longer a need to feed fears that can be dangerous when they have no real justification. If necessary, the doctor can prescribe the appropriate medications essential for the hot phase to proceed well.

If a cure is obtained, it is still a good idea to regularly return to consult the therapist to verify that there is no risk of the biological conflict reactivating. Work on discovering its psychic structure could be essential for one's personal evolution and for avoiding a recurrence of the illness. If the intense feeling is not found, the individual still has learned, in conversations with the therapist, that events and symptoms of the individual's present life can be the consequence of earlier events that he or she may have forgotten. Thus the patient acquires a new form of discernment that makes the patient the driver rather than the passenger of his or her own life. An illness will often transform different tissues of the same organ because the feeling of distress had several subtle shades. It is a good idea for the therapist to take these various nuances into consideration.

Resistances to Healing

Illnesses, misfortunes, and suffering prevent the patient from confronting the intolerable emotions that programmed them. Mountain climbers will not let go of one handhold until they are sure the next one will hold their weight. A change of beliefs beforehand (the creation of new handholds) is often necessary to finally be able to talk about the sources of profound suffering (letting go of the earlier handhold). The foundational dogmas of the family philosophy

("Money does not buy happiness," "One should not talk about sex," for example) can have perverse effects that require unmasking. When the individual is ready, he or she will progress and pass on to the next stage.

There are conflicts, however, whose resolution places the subject in a vicious circle that prevents the cure from taking place; this is known as chronicity (the state of being chronic or enduring for a long time).

Eczema is a phase in the repair of a conflict of separation. But kissing and touching the spouse with eczema may disgust the partner, and the person suffering from eczema again finds him- or herself alone. The sufferer then remanufactures a conflict and subsequent illness.

A symptom of a reparative phase that causes pain, and a lack of understanding of why it is happening, can also make an illness chronic: "My rheumatism"—the repair stage that follows a crisis of self-devaluation—"is so irritating that I will use it as another excuse to devalue my own worth."

There are biological and symbolic compensations that imprison the individual in his or her problem. For instance, when Mrs. Brown's husband abandoned her, this was a source of great distress for her. She became more masculine in appearance and behavior, a hormonal effect of her biological conflict of a feminine affective distress; she then grew fatter (an aggressive masculine reaction to abandonment). Given current ideas of what constitutes feminine beauty, she is then considered less alluring, and is unable to find a new partner. Feeling less and less attractive, she will increase in weight even more in order to catch the eye and become quite visible. Additinally, her weight gain is a life insurance policy when the winter of life is sensed and old age is a source of fear. Thus does she fall back on a perfectly archaic biological solution to take the place of the unresolved emotional issue. Given all of this, however, every time she weighs herself on the scale or looks in the mirror, she creates a conflict with her image and her silhouette, and she will try to diet again. This creates a vicious circle and the situation becomes frozen in place.

It may be in the patient's interest for the illness to continue (for example, being hard of hearing protects the patient from noise and what is connected to this noise, making it possible to not hear the other; paralysis allows the patient to find refuge from unpleasantness). Illness can be a means—sometimes the sole available means—to apply pressure to various people in our lives, to ensure their presence and compassion along with an additional spoonful of respect, attention, and even obedience. ("I took care of my mother for five years, and because you are my daughter, I want you to do the same for me.")

The illness can be maintained unconsciously because it establishes a link with the positive aspect (pleasant, valued memories) of the history preceding the DHS. For example: Sally's constipation began when, at her parent's request, she broke up with a young man. Now, more than forty years later, her constipation and the problems it has given her has allowed her to remain in touch with this beautiful love story from so long ago.

Illness also allows us to abandon our earlier goals without having to take responsibility for giving them up. It is the joker of the deck that permits us to discard the hand we are holding and have a good excuse to get out of the game. Illness can also serve as a trigger. It can act as a stimulus to action if we have not yet managed to take that first move to change our lives.

Someone who is seeking the healing of a cold illness is like a sailor who leaves the shore aboard a motorboat. The sailor is aware there is a point of no return. At what point will the boat no longer have enough gas to get back to land? To make this determination, the sailor takes stock of the fuel level and estimates the strength and direction of the winds, currents, tides, and waves. In similar fashion, we can ask if the energy reserves of a sick person are sufficient to repair the body and restore it to its "normal" state, so that once the person is cured, he or she can resume a normal life. Will someone nourishing a secret death wish try to arrange things so as to get past this point of no return?

Results

Since the time of these discoveries, thousands of people who believed their illnesses condemned them to death have been healed. Immediate cures are becoming increasingly numerous. The failures of men and women who, despite their belief, failed to find healing can be attributed to parameters that were neglected: the patient's decision to terminate discussions with the therapist, or simple human error.

The fault certainly does not lie in biology and the way it functions; it follows the same rules for all living things. There is life, and then there is what each of us makes of it. When the strictly science-based medicine of the present day has integrated these discoveries and abandoned some of its dogmas, the chances for healing will be greatly enhanced.

Faith, of course, is a very useful asset, if only for giving the individual the resolve to undertake this evolutionary approach and to follow through by setting up an appointment with a therapist. But it is even more useful in the reinforcement it gives the patient to seek, with that therapist, the information necessary to learn, throughout the time the body is undergoing repair, to avoid retriggering this conflict and all its attendant doubts. There are people who doubt their healing process because they do not have a clear understanding of the meaning of their illness. There are those who doubt their ability to change on their own and thus wait for others to change for them. Also, there are those whose doubts persist because of the intensity of their suffering. Yet others doubt because they do not get the comfort and support they need. And then there are people who believe their illness is a punishment from God. They do not give themselves permission to heal, as that would constitute putting more trust in their personal power than in God's authority. In short, there are doubts that can be lethal.

When a person is temporarily incapable of resolving a conflict, therefore, it may often be better to resort to the benefits offered by allopathic medicine.

This book is not a collection of miraculous healing stories. The tipping point in the healing of a person is a unique history (haven't you, the reader, already been healed naturally of some symptom at one or more times in your life?), whereas the way the brain and organs function is universal. I have taken what I believe to be the more sensible course of offering food for thought.

The therapists who practice this new discipline of life experience distinguish themselves by the speed with which they can unearth key information, and by the means they employ to find it (intuition, questionnaires, kinesiology, energy diagnostics, and so forth). While the energy body of humans is greatly affected by their emotions and by the defense strategies they have employed since childhood, I have not focused on energy work per se in this book. For those interested in furthering their understanding of energy work, I recommend books written by acupuncturists on this topic; they give the subject outstanding treatment.

The body's biology is One. There is only one way to get healed, by finding the correct information (it is a job for a detective), but numerous doorways exist that can provide access to this information and be the tipping point for the brain to heal. Homeopathy uses the doorway of the mouth, and with high dilutions of plants or minerals, it reveals the information of the concealed distress. Magnetism uses the doorway of the energetic body; acupuncture uses the doorway of the meridians and points; other traditional practitioners use other doorways or access various levels of brain function. Biological decoding, which uses the doorway of the ear and verbal exchange, seems to be the royal road to me, and the most effective today, enabling the cure of so-called "serious" diseases. Various doorways can be used as complements to each other.

The human concept of health is that of an asymptomatic state, but such a state can be unstable. When destiny and its timepiece make their demands, one of the ways to avoid straying too far from health is to view illness for what it really is: a survival system that invites one to evolve.

SIXTEEN

SOME HOPEFUL PERSPECTIVES

Happy is he who has found the secret causes of things.

VIRGIL, *The Georgics* II

You want healing?
Know first that your illness holds back your death . . .
You wish to attain your goal?
Know first that your destiny answers to the
    needs of your ancestors, point by point.

Today there are countless corporations that profit and prosper from the conflicts of human beings (arms merchants, legal firms, pharmaceutical manufacturers, religious sects, construction companies, and so forth), which ensures that these conflicts are given discreet support instead of being eradicated. Is it necessarily in the best interests of the extremely powerful pharmaceutical industry for biological decoding to make the prescription of its very, very costly chemotherapies more rare?

The dissemination of the biological discoveries that are capable of eliminating doubt, irrational fear, self-devaluation, and guilt will help humanity gradually emerge from the rut in which one individual is pitted against another. The corporations mentioned above will either evolve or disappear. Whatever efforts those seeking to prevent the spread of these discoveries may deploy, they are certain to be futile.

Throughout the world, researchers working in a large variety of different fields—some quite remote from the one examined here—are contributing findings to the medical community that confirm the significance of Dr. Hamer's discoveries. Humanity's thirst for knowledge will successfully lead to the journey's end, despite all the efforts made to prevent new wine from replacing the old. It is only a question of time.

Another Medical Culture

Not too many years from now, before people decide to visit a specialist for consultation, they will already have a healthy vision of what their symptoms truly represent, because biological laws, the meanings of illnesses, and the correlations between emotions and illnesses will have been taught to children at an elementary-school level. When an individual is given a diagnosis of cancer, the diagnosis will no longer create a conflict and thus aggravate the individual's condition. He or she will be ready to listen and consult without erecting mental barriers.

Doctors and therapists will guide patients to the tipping point of healing, and hospitals will guide and moderate the body's natural reparative functions when they present a danger to the patient. There will be fewer removals of organs, fewer chemical treatments, less emotional turmoil, and more warmth and empathetic feeling, which will create more truly enduring cures. The most deadly forms of endemic illnesses—malaria, for example—will also become increasingly rare.

The medical establishment will adopt lifesaving procedures congruent with the two-phase process of illness, and it will be possible to save lives that cannot be saved today. Rather than placing all hope for a cure in the discovery of new medicines, the doctor will instead go directly to the source—in other words, to the hidden emotion.

In Europe, a growing number of therapists are progressively integrating this subtle kind of aid, shedding light on family trees and their mysteries and, in the process, obtaining a more precise understanding of interpersonal relationships and healing. In increasing numbers, people are learning of the existence of biological laws and the metaphysics of illness. As a result, their lives can now continue to evolve properly, thanks to books, apprenticeships, consultations, and cures.

Should this lead us to conclude that illnesses themselves are potentially going to disappear?

An illness makes it possible to live within a given environment when an essential need has not been satisfied. Therefore illness is useful, and will remain so. Even when, thanks to evolution toward greater maturity and lucidity, illness has become rare, human beings will still have a need for it. It alone can prevent them from dying of shock when a major stress catches them by surprise. Is it possible to eradicate the unexpected on a planet that is experiencing constant evolution? No, but we can learn how to quickly disarm the mental and emotional conflicts caused by the unexpected events.

Being ill enables individuals to survive while in a state of conflict, and being able to survive enables them to continue to be of use to those who are close to them, their lines, and their societies.

In the future, if the new modality of healing known as "Biological Decoding" is adopted in full force, the duration and seriousness of the illnesses that today are considered impossible to avoid will diminish considerably. Operations on the physical organs of the body will still serve a purpose, but they too will be less frequent.

The new therapeutic modality will generate great savings in health expenditures. Expensive treatments "against" an illness will become increasingly rare. Because there will be fewer patients, less suffering, and less sophisticated medication, health insurance costs should fall well below current levels. In addition, it may be possible to reimburse patients for treatments that may, for some people, not be reimbursable today, such as psychotherapy, orthodontics, laser surgery, plastic surgery, and so forth. Every civilization has possessed treasures of knowledge that were overlooked by colonizers who found what could be converted into cash more attractive than the treasures of ancestral wisdom. Indigenous peoples the world over have abandoned excellent therapeutic and prophylactic systems to adopt the practices and beliefs of their colonizers. In this way, the dire remedies of one "occidental" culture have flooded other cultures, injecting values and beliefs that are destructive and disempowering.

Traditional Chinese medicine, as one example, has had to fight for its life against the pressures applied by Western lobbies. Homeopathy, despite its growing popularity and the increased numbers of practitioners who are trained in it, is a chief target of the pharmaceutical industry, which seeks to eliminate what it views as a dangerous rival.

Consultation with biogenealogists, biopsychogenealogists, and therapists specializing in Biological Decoding, whether they are licensed medical doctors or not, will become increasingly widespread and occasion no more notice than a visit to a doctor or a fortune-teller does today.

The Evolution of the Couple and the Family

If a couple is able to discover, before being married, the nature of the secret imperatives of both partners' ancestors and their unresolved problems, the two will undoubtedly have a better relationship. Love, like friendship, is built on a shared taste for betterment and for transcendence. How can we be available for this transcendence if some of our basic functions are unknown to us?

For couples who have witnessed a premature shift in their relationships, such as a loss of desire, perspectives from the standpoint of evolution that may now seem groundless will become quite real when the unconscious motivations that led the partners to join in the first place are revealed.

Those who have experienced happiness also share the desire to create healthy and happy descendants. Putting one's material affairs in order before dying is fine, but it is far better to resolve conflicts, make the acquaintance of one's family tree, write down one's personal history, and recount what one knows to one's descendants. To speak truthfully to one's children, telling them what was truly being felt at the moment of their conception, is a gift that will enable them to gain strength, health, and joy. Bringing one's own parents' histories into the open and sharing them with one's children and grandchildren will help them avoid hardship and difficulty.

A Common Underlying Belief Is on the Road to Extinction

Medicine, justice, and religion are all built on a common belief that has emerged from the old Persian concepts of the devil and of the existence of good and evil. This belief has led human beings to practice exclusion.

For example, leaders of religious sects declare that it is necessary to eliminate from the minds and hearts of humans the Evil One—Satan—whose expressions are humanity's instincts and its natural biological impulses.

Doctors have also taken part in shaping this belief with the idea that the ailing body could be corrupted by the Evil One, and they have exhausted themselves trying to remove malignant cells and abnormal functions by force to prevent them from corrupting the rest of the body.

Legislators and judges, for their part, have believed that the abnormal behaviors exhibited by certain members of a society were wicked and insane. They have isolated these individuals, or even killed them, so that they could not corrupt and disturb the entire society.

For a long time the Church of Rome fought the kings of Europe for political power. The church infiltrated the courts, influenced cabinet ministers, and associated closely with monarchs. Its dogmas and means of imposing a stable social order thus acquired greater influence. The abnormal, the marginal, the atypical—anything that might disturb the sweet routine of daily life—was "evil." Expelling it was a "duty." The idea of removing a cancerous organ or eliminating a symptom with a toxic medication, like the idea of isolating an individual in a psychiatric institution rather than searching for the cause of the problem and respecting its fruits, proceeded in neighborly fashion, supported by a philosophy that expected human beings to extract from their conduct all behaviors that created disorder. For a long time, medical schools were run by religious denominations; this goes a long way to explain why things are the way they are today.

With regard to legal practices, excluding from society the asocial individual, either by legally sanctioned murder or imprisonment, was the only response that people of greater privilege, deluded by visions of the immediate present, thought was viable.

In tomorrow's world, when we have abandoned these erroneous beliefs, the practices inherent in the disciplines of medicine, justice, and religion will evolve to more enlightened levels. The truth is that all of life is one; it is what it needs to be and what it should be—without the dualistic concepts of "good" versus "evil"—but instead with opposite forces that keep life in a proper homeostatic balance.

Does it make sense to think of centrifugal force as malignant and centripetal force as good? yin and yang are complimentary and opposite; neither of the two is evil *or* good.

The Disincarceration of Society

The number of psychiatric hospitals and prisons and the rates at which they are filled give clues to the level of maturity of a civilization. At the end of the second millennium, these isolation units were filled to capacity. By charging biochemists with the task of finding pharmaceutical solutions to behavioral disorders and by isolating mental patients, psychiatry, for lack of better ideas, has instituted a very subtle form of exclusion. This medication-based approach erects barriers that delay and defer the eruption of suffering. The discovery of the constellation of focal points in the brain makes it possible to cure a certain number of behavioral disorders and to envision the healing of all the others. The destiny of those detained in prisons or psychiatric hospitals might well improve.

Delinquency, like illness, has a meaning. In societies that define themselves by their conflicts, it provides a survival strategy for those who lack affection, love, and guidance. Delinquency is living proof of the hidden infamy of our societies, their secrets, their follies, their weaknesses, their doctrines and beliefs, and their fears. Antisocial actions, serious and deplorable as they may be, express the concealed history of one's close lineage and exhume ancestral conflicts and the illusions that nourished them.

Individuals do not become violent unless they have a program that directs them to behave in this fashion. People do not become thieves unless there is a history of theft in their family trees. Those condemned for violations of common law, terrorists or fanatics, or those interned for psychiatric reasons are all designated by their family trees to exhibit these behaviors. They are the links of the chain of their family tree that sacrifice themselves for the good of the line.

Individuals who aid former prisoners to reenter society know that there are few successful reintegrations. These efforts could be more successful if therapists specializing in deprogramming were systematically employed in such cases. In the long run, we can imagine an end to prisons altogether. What greater proof of a society's failure could there be but prisons?

Social health by means of imprisonment was the cynical utopian dream of a nineteenth-century Republican politician, as if imprisonment in cells of concrete and steel could help individuals make contact with their cellular memories and become better people. So why does man, who believes himself to be the most advanced and evolved creature of creation, put his fellows in prison? A little farther down the road that I am describing in this book, instead of prisons, there will be apple orchards.

In our recent judicial tradition, transgenerational programming has not been viewed as a factor. This has led to the current situation whereby one of two "actors" involved in a conflict receives punishment. The law punishes the "executioner" or assailant, whereas the "victim"—who, in fact, is not a victim by chance (as ancestral conflicts placed him or her into this position so that the true nature of the conflicts would be revealed)—is regarded as entirely innocent.

A victim always shares responsibility with the assailant for the event, but the victim does not know that. Something exists in the family tree of a victim that compelled the person to appear at a certain location at the same time as the assailant through the agency of an unconscious affinity, whether the assault be due to a rapist, human error, "bad luck," an airplane crash, an attack, or a natural catastrophe. Study of family memories and genealogical trees confirms this.

Such considerations naturally find themselves at the antipodes of the fashionable American philosophy that gives people the right to use the courts to attack their doctor or surgeon when an operation has failed, a tobacco company when smoking has caused a breathing disorder, or a fast-food chain when patronizing it has brought about chronic obesity. One thing is certain: as long as an individual transfers the responsibility (and that of his or her line) for a problem onto the shoulders of another person or persons, that individual is, at the same time, foreclosing on the possibility of a cure.

A mature society can arise only by virtue of individuals who are aware of their line's responsibility for what befalls them, and aware that they can act using their free will. Our societies currently violently condemn the marionette, but not the ancestral histories that are pulling the strings. True justice can be founded only on a deontology that takes into account this co-responsibility (which is also a co-irresponsibility). Humans are not lucid enough to pass judgment on their fellows. One day, thanks to biogenealogy, the word *prison* may be used so infrequently that it vanishes from the dictionaries.

More Love and Trust

How would it be possible to dislike people, those who are close to you in your daily life, when all the logic of their behaviors has been made visible? How could you hate your neighbors or your elders when you understand what kind of ancestral biological conflicts are motivating their behaviors? It will no longer be possible to fight ceaselessly with our nearest and dearest once we realize the impact that one lone, deeply felt emotion can have on the body.

With the advent of the practice of Biological Decoding, the longstanding habit of human societies to hunt out, a tangible individual to bear the blame, to be made the scapegoat, in the event of a "crime" or "disaster," will disappear. The microbe, the germ, the virus—guardian angels of the cells—will be cleansed of their guilt. And the human being will thus be deprived of one opportunity for self-devaluation, wherein an individual assumes the position of victim when confronted by the alleged violence of the microbial race.

The rehabilitation of microbes necessarily entails the revalorization of the invisible microbial portion of ourselves, which means our own revalorization and an assumption of our proper responsibilities. In the year 2000, thousands of perfectly healthy cows were incinerated because they were carriers of a prion protein molecule; and even today, millions of men and women across the planet are labeled, marginalized, isolated, and condemned because a hastily established dogma attributes a much greater danger to the HIV virus than it deserves.

Our political leaders will gain a greater awareness of the scope of their decisions thanks to an understanding of the first two biological laws, that of the powerful emotion that triggers the cold illness stage, and that of the resolution of the conflict, which triggers the hot reparative stage of the illness. The fear experienced by one generation will be transmuted into illnesses by the following generation. This is why all the alarmist "anti" campaigns in the affluent nations actually generate illnesses.

Knowledge of the phenomenon of transgenerational transmission will confer on humanity the ability to take action on the destiny of its descendants. It will awaken the minds of business people and politicians to a nontemporal planetary awareness and instruct them that time is space reiterated, and that the attitude of *après moi le deluge** is self-destructive.

How is it possible to be guilty of one thing when everything is the solution to everything else that is not our problem? How can we heal ourselves of our status as victims or executioners, and relinquish the habit of judgment, without a completely different understanding of life? What we are the least skilled in doing is

---

* This is a quote generally attributed to the French king Louis XV or, by some, to his mistress, Madame de Pompadour. The literal meaning is, "After me, the flood." Its more accessible meaning would be: "What matters is me right now, the future and other people have no importance for me."

passing judgment, for when we judge another person, we are actually projecting onto the other, out of a need to reassure ourselves, the delirious and insane ideas that have been spawned in the obscurity of the family and the social imagination.

Political ideology has broken down at the side of the road. It is waiting for a new kind of fuel, a totally new energy that is neither right nor left. We have all inherited a fear of the irrational. Do not even the strongest among us have our superstitious moments? When this fear vanishes, it will be possible for us to heal from our collective delusions.

No social plan of any duration can be crafted today as long as mindless beliefs (the germ is wicked, the aberrant and cancerous cell is insane, nature is crazy, the Evil One is tempting humankind, and so on) are maintained by sects, lobbies, and/or political parties. How can we see the harmony of the world if we continue to wear distorting lenses over our eyes?

Wage War with Love

If the principle of war is natural and biologically encoded to defend one's territory or to conquer new territories, the practice of war between humans should look like battles between animals of the same species. Yet rare is it that animals of the same species slaughter one another. Humans, curiously enough, have forgotten (since arms dealers first appeared?) that it is possible to war with their peers without having the ritual end in death and suffering.

The defeated wolf exposes his throat, and the victor looks away.

Genocidal crusades legitimized by a belief in the existence of good and evil have conditioned human beings to forget the biological purpose of combat. The old stag that rebukes the young pretender seeking to dethrone him in order to become the leader of the herd does not try to kill his opponent, even after hours of combat.

Outside of the animal kingdom, only the children of human beings, in the ritual battles they engage in during playtime, still know that war can be waged with love, in compliance with the archetypes of interdependent combat, in stimulated classes for survival school.

In every way, and in the final analysis, it is always the soft that wears away the hard. The teeth on the harrow of the cultivator wear away from scratching furrows into the soil, although the ground is much less hard than the steel from which these teeth are made. It is not the most aggressive people with the strongest weapons and the best armor who win, nor is it the most rigid and totalitarian of philosophies that triumphs. Rather, it is the flexibility of human beings, their mobility, their adaptability—in short, their capacity for love—that always eventually prevails. A growing sensitivity to the biological functions of life will enable a change to take place in the hearts of human beings. We all want, without exception, mornings that make us want to rise up and sing. We all want to experience hearts overfilled with joy. We need to climb back, like the salmon, to the source of our conflicts before we form ourselves into armed battalions.

In whose interest is it to draw up more plans for war? War begins with the second rifle shot, according to the sage. And the victor is the one who can go beyond the spirit of discord.

Individuals are to the universe what cells are to the body of the individual. When human beings kill other human beings, the world creates a depression. The illusion of separation prevents us from seeing that all are one in service to the great cosmic whole. Inside any living being every cell has a purpose; there is not a single one that is superfluous or of more importance than another. Inside the earth/universe body, no individual is of any greater importance than another.

Has anyone ever witnessed bone cells marching off to war against muscle or hepatic cells? No. Rejecting a black human being, a yellow human being, a human being whose skin color has been made darker by the environment, is the same as refusing to accept and maintain the black, yellow, and tanned cells of one's own body. It is a demand for an undifferentiating environment and thus undifferentiated cells—in other words, cancerous cells. One day men will know how, like their cousins the animals, to wage war without killing, and without destroying nature.

Agenda

Every morning when we stand in front of the mirror, we can see that we look very much as we did the day before. Our face and body still bear a strong resemblance to what they looked like a year ago. However, in the space of that year, a large number of our cells are no longer the same; they have been renewed. This cellular renewal is something we often forget is taking place when we do not have wounds, intense emotional shocks, or illnesses to remind us. And because we forget about it, we easily underestimate the body's ability to heal itself. Cannot this morning ritual of standing in front of the mirror be an opportunity to touch base with this discreet but permanent renewal?

Illness is a potential meeting between the normal individual, in a state of good health, and his or her super (wo)man side. Thanks to illness, individuals can gain awareness of all the plans contained in their genes and then discover the extent of their powers to adapt. Thanks to illness, individuals gain access to the trials and ordeals experienced by all their ancestors, both near and remote.

Without this privileged moment, in which the genes give expression to something completely different than what they normally express, individuals have no awareness of their line and what it has experienced, and thus grow isolated from it.

Physical pain automatically accompanies numerous repairs of the body, such as during their consolidating and scarring phases; during these times, movement and agitation can be dangerous.

Only pain can truly force a person to stay still. Pain can be the herald of healing, but it can also indicate that physiological limits have been reached. It teaches humility and forces one to rest, as if one were a plant rather than an animal or human. It can prevent the dangerous enthusiastic overreaction that could give birth to unbridled ambition or a state of unawareness, with lethal consequences. It reminds us that we still have conflicts to resolve. It is a valuable rendezvous with our physiobiological needs and an opportunity to see the admirable perfection of nature that was clever enough to invent edema to render aid to parts of the body that have suffered a trauma.

The cold phase of the illness has a rendezvous with the hot phase that brings about its disappearance, just like the meeting of the opposites yin and yang, of light and darkness, of acid and alkaline, which create the conditions without which life would be impossible.

The unavoidable rendezvous with death is a central piece to the puzzle of human function and behavior. Because death is dreaded so pathologically by many, they cling all the more tenaciously to life. This increases the excessive stress that initially brought about the life-threatening situation and increases its intensity.

When it comes to the subject of death, the human imagination has manufactured, in the absence of any scientific information on the phenomenon, a large number of dogmas (heaven and hell, reincarnation, and so forth). But doctors and those who have had near-death experiences may have much to teach us. Illness could well be a rendezvous with our fears and the illusions that feed them.

Today it appears that information has or would have eternal life. The ability of a piece of information to be memorized and transmitted, in whatever physical medium, guarantees the existence of an "after" following death. Transgenerational programming carries much evidence of the persistent nature of this impalpable set of data that characterizes an individual (and the individual's relationships with those around him or her), since that same set can be found anew in some of the individual's descendants. Thus it is that the dead have a rendezvous with the living.

Humans live their lives apart from their family trees and their pasts. They live lives separate from their fellows, to the extent they can even find themselves in conflict or in competition. May this book, whose main theme is life, serve as an opportunity to make a rendezvous with the sensation of unity! The sense of union is capable of erasing even the most recurrent conflicts. Humans distinguish themselves from plants and animals by their ability to think intentionally and independently. This gives them the power to disarm their biological conflicts.

The Earth Still Turns Around the Sun

From the dawn of time, living organisms have amassed strategies in their genes and bequeathed them to new generations. Evolution has not ended; we are all mutants. If, by eliminating the gene of an illness, the only thing that is accomplished is a transfer of energy to another organ, all that is happening is the creation of another kind of illness.

Be this as it may, the idea of finding procedures for altering chromosomes has seduced corporate entities in search of new products. The allopathic nano-medicines currently in preparation (nano-probes, dendrimeres, nano-diagnostic tools, nano-therapies, artificial white corpuscles, targeted destruction systems of cancerous cells, and so forth), masterworks of human genius, will offer a slight degree of progress in comparison to today's allopathic methods and practices, but will end in results that are little different from those we can obtain today. With the exception of some extremely useful prosthetic devices for eyes (artificial retinas, for example), ears, and other areas of the body, and some new therapeutic gadgets, this medicine will still be an "anti" medicine. It will not eradicate the cause of disease and will treat patients precariously, with no thought to their emotional past or family tree, thus making them dependent on costly and repeated treatments.

By causing the disappearance of symptoms by force and by ruse, individuals spoil the opportunity they have been given to change what is not working in their lives. The guardrail of the symptom is replaced by the anguish of remaining ill. If human beings are one day transformed into robots from within, genetically modified, manipulated, and standardized, how will they manage excessive distress? What steps will the androids take to know who they truly are?

Associations and governments alike are militating today for universal healthcare, and demanding price reductions in medications and the fall of patents into the public domain. I invite them to experience another belief instead, to discover the meaning of illnesses and, through that, discover the therapeutic means accessible to everyone—from the depths of Burundi to the Mexican deserts—with no need for expensive pills or cumbersome infrastructures.

My objective is to demonstrate that it is possible to look at illness and destiny in a new way that can offer both salvation and healing. Sickness is to the living being what the balancing pole is to a tightrope walker. Do you dare set off on the cord of your life stretching from birth to death without a balancing pole?

Tomorrow, new discoveries will come to enrich this therapy of Biological Decoding, as the study of the brain is still in its infancy. Other books, containing new knowledge, will appear to awaken the wisdom that slumbers inside every one of us.

SUGGESTED READING
AND RESOURCES

Suggested Reading

Gérard Athias. *Racines familiales de la "mal a dit"*. [The Family Roots of Illness.] France: Pictorus, 2002.

Boris Cyrulnik. *Les vilains petits canards*. [Ugly Ducklings.] France: Odile Jacob, 2004.

Régis Dutheil and Brigitte Dutheil. *L'homme superlumineux*. [The Superluminous Man.] France: Sand & Tchou, 2003.

Eric Edelmann. *Jésus parlait araméen*. [Jesus Spoke Aramaic.] France: Du Relié, 2000.

Jean-Paul Escande and Claire Escande. *Biologies*. France: Empecheurs Penser en Rond, 1997.

Christian Flèche. *Mon corps pour me guérir, Le décodage biologique des maladies*. [My Body Can Heal Me: The Biological Decoding of Illness.] Barret-sur-Meouge, France: Le Souffle d'Or, 2005.

———. *Le Roy se crée, Conte métaphorique en décodage biologique*. [The King Creates Himself: Metaphorical Stories of Biological Decoding.] Barret-sur-Meouge, France: Le Souffle d'Or, 2002.

Christian Flèche and Jean Jacques Lagardet. *L'instant de la guérison.* [The Moment of Healing.] Barret-sur-Meouge, France: Le Souffle d'Or, 2004.

Didier Grandgeorges. *Homéopathie, chemin de vie.* [Homeopathy: A Way of Life.] France: Edicomm, 1999.

Robert Guinee. *Les maladies, mémoires de l'evolution.* [Diseases, Memories of Evolution.] Brussels, Belgium: Amyris, 2004.

Ryck Geerd Hamer. *Summary of the New Medicine.* Genova, Italy: Amici di Dirk, 2000.

Elisabeth Horowitz. *Se libérer du destin familial.* [Freedom from Your Family Destiny.] Paris, France: Dervy, 2000.

———. *Sous l'influence du destin familial: John Fitzgerald Kennedy et les programmations secrètes de l'arbre généalogique.* [Under the Influence of Family Destiny: John Fitzgerald Kennedy and the Secret Programmings of the Family Tree.] Paris, France: Dervy, 2003.

Arthur Janov. *Imprints: The Lifelong Effects of the Birth Experience.* New York: Coward-McCann, 1983.

———. *The Biology of Love.* Amherst, NY: Prometheus Books, 2000.

Pierre-Jean Thomas Lamotte. *Écouter et comprendre la maladie.* [Listen to and Understand Disease.] Paris, France: Éditions Téqui, 2002.

Ernest L. Rossi. *Psychobiology of Mind-Body Healing.* New York: W. W. Norton, 1993.

Jacques Ruffié. *Le sexe at la mort.* [Sex and Death.] France: Odile Jacob, 2000.

Hervé and Mireille Scala. *Des ancêtres encombrants? Se réconcilier avec son histoire familiale.* [Burdensome Ancestors? Reconcile with Your Family History.] Barret-sur-Meouge, France: Le Souffle d'Or, 2004.

Salomon Sellam. *Le syndrome du gisant.* [The Syndrome of Lying.] France: Bérangel, 2005.

Bernard Vial and Biondetta Mandrant. *La médecine affective au jardin.* [Effective Medicine from the Garden.] France: Similia, 1996.

Resources

www.newmedicine.ca

Dr. Ryke Geerd Hamer's official English Web site. Contains the most recent developments in Biological Decoding.

www.germannewmedicine.ca

Includes information for practitioners and patients and an introduction to Dr. Hamer's Five Biological Laws of German New Medicine.

www.medicinasagrada.com/plan-en.html

A Web site put together by a pair of Biological Decoding practitioners in Quebec. Contains information on workshops and conferences.

www.biodecoding.com

Web site of the Institute of Biodecoding, founded in the United States in 2003 by Marie-Anne Boularand.

INDEX

INDEX